COUPLES COPING WITH STRESS

Emerging Perspectives on Dyadic Coping

Edited by Tracey A. Revenson,
Karen Kayser, and Guy Bodenmann

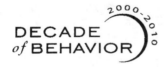

American Psychological Association • Washington, DC

Published by
American Psychological Association
750 First Street, NE
Washington, DC 20002
www.apa.org

To order
APA Order Department
P.O. Box 92984
Washington, DC 20090-2984
Tel: (800) 374-2721; Direct: (202) 336-5510
Fax: (202) 336-5502; TDD/TTY: (202) 336-6123
Online: www.apa.org/books/
E-mail: order@apa.org

In the U.K., Europe, Africa, and the Middle East, copies may be ordered from
American Psychological Association
3 Henrietta Street
Covent Garden, London
WC2E 8LU England

Typeset in Century Schoolbook by Nova Graphic Services, Jamison, PA

Printer: Victor Graphics, Inc., Baltimore, MD
Cover Designer: Mercury Publishing Services, Rockville, MD
Technical/Production Editor: Emily Leonard

The opinions and statements published are the responsibility of the authors, and such opinions and statements do not necessarily represent the policies of the American Psychological Association.

Library of Congress Cataloging-in-Publication Data

Couples coping with stress : emerging perspectives on dyadic coping / edited by Tracey A. Revenson, Karen Kayser, and Guy Bodenmann.
       p. cm. — (Decade of behavior) (APA science volumes)
   Includes bibliographical references and index.
   ISBN 1-59147-204-0 (alk. paper)
  1. Marital psychotherapy. 2. Couples. 3. Stress (Psychology) 4. Adjustment (Psychology)
I. Revenson, Tracey A. II. Kayser, Karen. III. Bodenmann, Guy. IV. Series. V. Series: APA science volumes

  RC488.5.C64343 2005
  616.89'1562—dc22

                                                2004020293

British Library Cataloguing-in-Publication Data
A CIP record is available from the British Library.

Printed in the United States of America
First Edition

To Richard S. Lazarus,
whose creativity and ideas influenced
the work of all the authors in this book.

APA Science Volumes

APA Decade of Behavior Volumes

Contents

Contributors

Ana F. Abraído-Lanza, PhD, Mailman School of Public Health, Columbia University, New York, NY

Linda K. Acitelli, PhD, Department of Psychology, University of Houston, Houston, TX

Hoda J. Badr, PhD, Department of Behavioral Science, M. D. Anderson Cancer Center, University of Texas, Houston

Chris Barker, PhD, Sub-Department of Clinical Health Psychology, University College London, London, England

Guy Bodenmann, PhD, Institute for Family Research and Counseling, University of Fribourg, Fribourg, Switzerland

Thomas N. Bradbury, PhD, Department of Psychology, University of California—Los Angeles

Linda Charvoz, PhD, Institute for Family Research and Counseling, University of Fribourg, Fribourg, Switzerland

Annette Cina, PhD, Institute for Family Research and Counseling, University of Fribourg, Fribourg, Switzerland

Carolyn E. Cutrona, PhD, Institute for Social and Behavioral Research and Department of Psychology, Iowa State University, Ames

Anita DeLongis, PhD, University of British Columbia, Department of Psychology, Vancouver, Canada

Kelli A. Gardner, MS, Institute for Social and Behavioral Research and Department of Psychology, Iowa State University, Ames

Caren Jordan, PhD, Department of Psychology, East Carolina University, Greenville, NC

Benjamin R. Karney, PhD, Department of Psychology, University of Florida, Gainesville

Karen Kayser, PhD, Graduate School of Social Work, Boston College, Chestnut Hill, MA

S. Deborah Majerovitz, PhD, Department of Political Science and Psychology, York College, The City University of New York, New York, NY

Melady Preece, PhD, Department of Psychology, University of British Columbia, Vancouver, Canada

Nancy Pistrang, PhD, Sub-Department of Clinical Health Psychology, University College London, London, England

Tracey A. Revenson, PhD, Social-Personality Psychology, The Graduate Center of The City University of New York, New York, NY

Daniel W. Russell, PhD, Department of Human Development and Family Studies, Iowa State University, Ames

Shachi Shantinath, PhD, Institute for Family Research and Counseling, University of Fribourg, Fribourg, Switzerland

Lisa B. Story, MS, Department of Psychology, University of California—Los Angeles

Kathrin Widmer, PhD, Institute for Family Research and Counseling, University of Fribourg, Fribourg, Switzerland

Foreword

In early 1988, the American Psychological Association (APA) Science Directorate began its sponsorship of what would become an exceptionally successful activity in support of psychological science—the APA Scientific Conferences program. This program has showcased some of the most important topics in psychological science and has provided a forum for collaboration among many leading figures in the field.

The program has inspired a series of books that have presented cutting-edge work in all areas of psychology. At the turn of the millennium, the series was renamed the Decade of Behavior Series to help advance the goals of this important initiative. The Decade of Behavior is a major interdisciplinary campaign designed to promote the contributions of the behavioral and social sciences to our most important societal challenges in the decade leading up to 2010. Although a key goal has been to inform the public about these scientific contributions, other activities have been designed to encourage and further collaboration among scientists. Hence, the series that was the "APA Science Series" has continued as the "Decade of Behavior Series." This represents one element in APA's efforts to promote the Decade of Behavior initiative as one of its endorsing organizations. For additional information about the Decade of Behavior, please visit http://www.decadeofbehavior.org.

Over the course of the past years, the Science Conference and Decade of Behavior Series has allowed psychological scientists to share and explore cutting-edge findings in psychology. The APA Science Directorate looks forward to continuing this successful program and to sponsoring other conferences and books in the years ahead. This series has been so successful that we have chosen to extend it to include books that, although they do not arise from conferences, report with the same high quality of scholarship on the latest research.

We are pleased that this important contribution to the literature was supported in part by the Decade of Behavior program. Congratulations to the editors and contributors of this volume on their sterling effort.

Steven J. Breckler, PhD
Executive Director for Science

Virginia E. Holt
*Assistant Executive Director
for Science*

Preface

In a *New Yorker* book review, Rebecca Mead (2003) cited John Milton's *Doctrine and Discipline of Divorce* (1643), in which he instructs Parliament that "In God's intention, a meet and happy conversation is the chiefest and noblest end of marriage" (p. 80). Mead suggested that by *conversation* Milton meant much more than the "marital chatter about school districts or visits to the in-laws" . . . or even the familiar, forlorn spousal inquiry, "What are you thinking about?" (p. 80). On the contrary, we take Milton's use of the word *conversation* on its face. These small everyday concerns, worries, and challenges are the stuff of which marriages, and more specifically marital coping, are made.

This volume addresses the construct of *dyadic coping* between people in intimate relationships. By strict definition, dyadic coping involves both partners and is the interplay between the stress signals of one partner and the coping reactions of the other or a genuine act of common (shared) coping. As the chapters in this volume illustrate, the construct of dyadic coping is nuanced, interpreted differently by the chapter authors to include processes such as everyday communication, interpersonal conflict, joint problem solving, the giving and receiving of emotional support, and dealing with life stressors as a *we* not just two *I*s. We are excited to share innovative conceptualizations and cutting-edge research on dyadic coping in this book.

This volume emerged from two international conferences on stress and coping processes among couples organized by Guy Bodenmann of the University of Fribourg, Switzerland, and Karen Kayser of Boston College, Massachusetts. In 1999, Bodenmann and Kayser had started collaborative work on dyadic coping and realized the need for scientific exchange among scholars working on these issues from different perspectives. The first invited conference, held in Fribourg, Switzerland, on September 18–19, 2000, was dedicated to this idea and provided an excellent platform. A small group of well-known researchers who had been working in the area of stress and coping in couples was brought together for 3 intensive days of presentation, discussion, and critique. Researchers came from Austria, Canada, Germany, Italy, Switzerland, and the United States. The conference was particularly successful in that it brought together researchers from different psychological traditions (close relationships, marital therapy, and health psychology) and whose scholarly networks had had only minimal contact to that point. A clear consensus at the end of the conference was that many ideas had only been touched on and that the group needed to continue working together to refine the notion of dyadic coping and its application to clinical practice. A second conference was held in Chestnut Hill, Massachusetts, at Boston College on October 12–14, 2002. With funding from the Science Directorate of the American Psychological Association (APA), the circle of presenters and discussants was enlarged and a small "audience" participated in the discussions as well.

The primary aim of this book is to present current approaches on stress and coping in couples, to bring American and European contributions together, and to stimulate further fruitful scientific exchange on this topic of growing importance. Intended primarily for scholars in the field of marital research, stress and coping research, and interpersonal relationships, the book also serves as a useful reader for practitioners. As the idea of dyadic coping is a new and innovative approach in the area of marital therapy, this volume should be of interest to therapists as well.

Although the conference attendees raised the idea of a collaborative publication at the first conference, it was not until the APA Science Directorate became involved that this book became a reality. We thank the APA Science Directorate and Boston College for funding the 2002 conference that started the seed of this book germinating. We also would like to thank Michelle Taylor of Boston College for coordinating the 2002 Boston Conference, Deborah McCall of the APA Science Directorate for assisting us with the conference planning, Mary Lynn Skutley and Phuong Huynh of APA Books for shepherding us through the publication process, Kate Silfen for her careful editing, and Adeane Bregman for her diligent research on the artwork for the book. We thank Alberto Godenzi, Dean of the Boston College Graduate School of Social Work, who generously released Karen Kayser from her teaching responsibilities to work on the conference. We are grateful to Michael Smyer, Associate Vice President for Research at Boston College, for his encouragement and support for the conference on which this book is based. We also thank all of the authors of the chapters for their cooperative and engaged work (and willingness to write quickly) and their contributions to this book. We would like to thank Linda Roberts for her thorough review and helpful critique of the book manuscript. Most important, we thank the other half of our own couples: Edward Seidman, Fred Groskind, and Corinne Bodenmann helped us cope with putting this book together while enjoying all the stresses and pleasures of married life (of which our children Molly Revenson; Emma Groskind; and Arliss, Aimée, and Ruben Bodenmann are a large part). And finally, thanks to Kit Kittredge and Molly McIntyre, whose images kept the first two authors sane during the summer of 2003 as they juggled their own American girls and editing this book.

Reference

Mead, R. (2003, August 11). Love's labors: Monogamy, marriage, and other menaces. *The New Yorker,* pp. 80–81.

COUPLES COPING
WITH STRESS

Introduction

Tracey A. Revenson, Karen Kayser, and
Guy Bodenmann

Over the past 30 years, the lion's share of research on stress and coping has focused almost exclusively on the coping efforts used by *individuals,* describing types or modes of coping strategies and their effects on physical and mental health outcomes. Major life stressors do not limit their influence to individuals but instead spread out like crabgrass to affect the lives of others in the individual's social network: family, friends, coworkers, neighbors, and even whole communities. Quite simply, people cope in the context of relationships with others. And those "others" are affected by the same stressors in a pattern of radiating effects (Kelly, 1971). Yet relatively few coping researchers have investigated how intimate partners cope with stress *as a couple* or how the coping efforts of partners mutually influence each other. It seems that an essential step toward further clarification of the relationship between stress and health involves examining coping as it naturally occurs within the context of significant relationships, in particular, the marital or marital-type relationship.

The past decade has witnessed the development of several theoretical frameworks for studying how couples cope together with life stress. Whereas there were only a few contributions published on stress and coping in couples before the 1990s, an increasing amount of theoretical and empirical work on this topic has emerged in the last decade (see Fig. 1). A number of researchers, primarily in the United States and Western Europe, became interested in how coping research could move past the individual level to

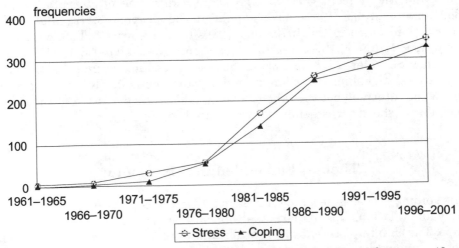

Figure 1. Growth in publications on stress and coping among couples over a 40-year period.

3

include the family context and began developing theoretical frameworks, empirical research, and innovative practice models to address these issues.

These developments surfaced at a time in our social history when stress permeates Western society and radical social changes challenge couples and families. For example, the dramatic increase in women working outside the home has led to juggling of work and family life (Artis & Pavalko, 2003; Crosby & Jaskar, 1993; Shelton & John, 1996). The likelihood of becoming a caregiver for an older family member who has a chronic mental or physical health condition is increasing for both women and men and has led to the type of stress known as *caregiver burden* (Marks, 1996; Marks, Lambert, & Choi, 2002; Schulz, O'Brien, Bookwala, & Fleissner, 1995). Economic stressors and strains have pushed many couples to increase their work hours in order to maintain a lifestyle promoted by the larger culture. Daily fears of terrorism and violence ranging from urban crime to political conflicts, wars, and ethnic clashes, are present worldwide.

Coupled with this multiplicity of daily and chronic stressors are the dwindling resources in our social environment to deal with them. Almost every form of social capital has been on the decrease (Putnam, 2000). As these resources become less available in the larger society, more pressure is placed on intimate partners and family members to deal with the stresses of daily life. Without the coping abilities and skills to manage the stress, many couple relationships suffer or break down. Karney, Story, and Bradbury (see chap. 1, this volume) suggest that this inability to cope with stress, coupled with poverty and low social resources, is a key reason for the high divorce rate in Western countries. At the very least, we know it is a fundamental and ubiquitous reason for seeking counseling and psychotherapy.

A major critique of stress and coping theories is that coping is not an individual process but occurs within a social and historical context (Revenson, 2003). Newer theoretical approaches such as *relationship-focused coping* (Coyne & Fiske, 1992), interpersonal *regulatory processes* (DeLongis & O'Brien, 1990; O'Brien & DeLongis, 1997), *coping congruence* (Revenson, 1994, 2003) and the *systemic-transactional conceptualization of stress and coping* (Bodenmann, 1995, 1997) have expanded the original stress and coping theories laid down in the 1970s and 1980s (e.g., Lazarus & Folkman, 1984; Lazarus & Launier, 1978; Pearlin, Lieberman, Menaghan, & Mullan, 1981; Pearlin & Schooler, 1978) and bring the notion of coping within the context of intimate relationships to the foreground. Dyadic coping involves both partners and is the interplay between the stress signals of one partner and the coping reactions of the other, a genuine act of shared coping.

Themes Embedded in this Volume

This volume presents new approaches in stress and coping research that focus on dyadic relationships, in particular, marital or long-term intimate relationships. The chapters present theoretical frameworks, formative research to test those frameworks, and translation of research findings into practice principles. *Emerging perspectives*, the phrase used in the book's subtitle, captures the character of the scholarship presented in this volume. Although the scholarship is original and at times pathbreaking, it is not always fully developed or without logical flaws. A first effort to assemble ideas that bridge several disciplines and two continents is bound to seem provisional. Definitions of *dyadic coping* differ from chapter to chapter, for example. Thus, the collection of perspectives in this volume creates a somewhat dizzying array of overlapping conceptualizations rather than a single cohesive conceptual model that is ready to be widely applied. We hope that this volume serves as a necessary first step to move the scholarship toward a heightened awareness of points of convergence and divergence and toward more integrative models to be tested.

Five prominent themes described below emerge from the individual chapters and are woven through the volume.

Conceptual Frameworks for Dyadic Coping Must Be Dyadic

Almost all the chapters have something to say about the conceptual underpinnings of dyadic coping processes: What should we be looking for? These conceptual issues frame the questions that are asked in couples research and point to methodologies that are needed to answer "couple-level" questions. Most importantly the dyad, or relationship, should be the unit of analysis at all stages of the research process, from conceptualizing the problem through methods and measurement to data analyses and interpretation. Conceptualization of the pattern of coping between two people—in Lazarus' terms, the person–environment transaction (Lazarus & Launier, 1978)—is the essential beginning of couples research. Obtaining data from both partners indicates progress in recognizing the limitations of individual constructions of coping, but collecting data from both partners does not in and of itself constitute dyadic-level research. Several chapters in this book (see chaps. 1, 3, & 7) illustrate how analyses at multiple levels of analysis can be utilized to reveal dyadic or couple-level coping.

Know Thy Stressor

A second theme is how the nature of the stressor affects dyadic coping processes. Literally hundreds of studies have shown that the properties of stressors shape coping efforts and adaptation (Cohen, Kessler, & Gordon, 1997). These properties include the magnitude of the stressor (minor stressors such as daily hassles or small life events vs. major stressors); the duration and nature of stress exposure (acute, intermittent, repeated, or chronic); the domain of stress (work, family, or medical); and the stressor's radiating effects on other stressors (i.e., stress contagion). The first chapter of this book, by Karney and his colleagues, emphasizes the distinction between acute versus chronic stressors as they affect marital quality among newlyweds. In chapter 3, Preece and DeLongis illustrate the confluence and reciprocal influences of major and minor stresses within the realm of stepparenting. Other chapters focus on single major life stressors, such as chronic or life-threatening illness (see chaps. 5, 6, & 7, this volume), depression (see chap. 5, this volume), and the transition to parenthood (see chap. 5, this volume).

Dyadic Coping With Stress Is a Process

Apart from the differentiation of the various forms of stress, it is critical to capture the dynamics of the coping process (Lazarus & Launier, 1978; Pearlin et al., 1981). The experience of dyadic-level stress in couples is a process of mutual influence in which the stress of one partner affects the other if the partners' coping skills (independently and jointly) are not sufficient to handle the stressor. It also makes sense to distinguish different phases within the stress and coping process and to assess stress and coping on multiple levels (individual and partner) within a specific social context. Bodenmann (see chap. 2, this volume) proposes an integrative framework for studying dyadic stress that is useful for both planning research and understanding different coping processes in intimate relationships. Several chapters (e.g., chaps. 5, 8, & 9, this volume) use a similar model of dyadic coping for understanding marital interactions under stress and developing innovative interventions and treatments.

We should note that although all the contributors share a general framework of dyadic-level coping, the chapters in this volume constitute "variations on a theme." Moreover, this volume is the first to present most of the current models of dyadic coping in one place. It is intriguing to see how many different models of dyadic coping are proposed and how each one captures a slightly different perspective. For example, Cutrona and her coauthors (see chap. 4, this volume) emphasize interpersonal trust as both a predictor of and component of dyadic coping; whereas Revenson and her coauthors (see chap. 7, this volume), Acitelli and Badr (see chap. 6, this volume), and Preece and DeLongis (see chap. 3, this volume) focus more on the *fit* or congruence between partners' coping and how it operates within the larger social context of family.

Dyadic Coping Within an Interpersonal Framework

The fourth theme emphasizes the interdependence of the constructs of coping and social support. Specifically, the success of coping efforts is heavily determined by others' responses. Although coping and support are overlapping concepts, they are not indistinguishable and each offers something unique to the understanding of human adaptation (see chap. 2, this volume). Moreover, it is important to separate social support transactions with persons outside of the marriage or dyadic unit from those with the spouse or partner. Both are essential components of dyadic coping processes, but are quite different. Almost all the chapters in this volume explore the mechanisms by which dyadic coping facilitates the exchange of social support and how social support processes influence coping processes. Some chapters focus on the broad concept of support provision as it affects marital quality (see chap. 4, this volume) or adaptation to major stress (see chap. 7, this volume); whereas others focus on interpersonal communication processes (see chaps. 5 & 6, this volume).

Translating Research Into Intervention

A final theme of this volume is the translation of dyadic-coping research into psychosocial interventions. Although the last section is devoted to intervention research on dyadic coping, applications to practice are emphasized throughout all of the chapters. The applications are illustrated in clinical work with individual couples (see chaps. 5 & 9, this volume) as well as more comprehensive interventions for couples facing marital distress (see chap. 8, this volume).

Content and Organization

This book is organized into three parts. The first part, "The Role of Stress in Dyadic Coping Processes," begins our examination of the concept of dyadic stress, its effect on couples' coping processes and relationship outcomes, and theoretical frameworks used to study dyadic coping processes. In chapter 1, Karney, Story, and Bradbury use longitudinal data on newly married couples to investigate the differential effects of acute and chronic stress on marital outcomes. Often the role of the external environment is overlooked as researchers focus primarily on the internal working of the couple's relationship and not its context. These authors offer a new perspective on understanding stress and use a multilevel methodology to systematically answer the question, "What kinds of negative outcomes are predicted by what kinds of stress?"

In chapter 2, Bodenmann expands on the concept of dyadic stress and coping with an innovative and dynamic theory of the dyadic coping process. He presents a typology of dyadic coping that distinguishes both positive and negative forms. This theory is supported by empirical findings on more than 1,000 couples, using multiple methods of data collection and various research designs. He investigates the questions, "How does stress affect marriage?" and "How does dyadic coping affect the relationship between stress and marital quality?"

Preece and DeLongis (chap. 3) expand interpersonal stress and coping to the rich context of stepfamilies. They examine how couples in stepfamilies use five coping strategies to manage interpersonal stressors and report findings on the connection between coping and relationship quality between parents and children. A unique feature of their research is the focus on both short-term (i.e., within the course of a single day) and long-term predictors (i.e., across 2 years) of relationship quality in stepfamilies. The authors illustrate how multilevel models can assist with the methodological problems that challenge researchers studying these complex systems of stepfamilies.

The second part of this book, "Social Support, Dyadic Coping, and Interpersonal Communication," contains chapters that focus on the interplay between dyadic coping and social support processes. In chapter 4, Cutrona, Russell, and Gardner present a model of relationship enhancement in which they explain how social support enhances health and well-being within the context of intimate relationships. They grapple with the question of how social support influences health and bring to light a neglected mechanism in the process through which supportive acts influence health: interpersonal trust. Drawing on both experimental and longitudinal naturalistic studies of couples, the authors offer compelling evidence for the interactions among social support, attributions, and trust. For the practitioner, they offer valuable suggestions for interventions and assessment of social support in intimate relationships. The chapter provides a new perspective on the long-range implications of how well or poorly couples support each other during difficult times—both for the relationship and health and well-being of each partner.

Pistrang and Barker (chap. 5) take the study of social support to a micro-level of analysis as they examine partners' responses during conversations of helping interactions. Using a narrative approach, they untangle partners' communication processes as they cope with serious stresses, including breast cancer and the transition to parenthood. Their study provides a unique dimension to this volume, in that the analysis focuses intensively on conversational analysis and has direct application to preventive therapy for couples. In their role as therapist researchers, Pistrang and Barker extend more conventional narrative approaches to what they describe as a *tape-assisted recall method* in which the partners are asked to review their own conversations and identify moments of empathy and lack of empathy and provide alternatives for communication. This communication analysis is embedded in a broader discussion of why social support is important for couples under stress, how this particular approach fills some gaps in the communication and psychotherapy literatures, and how an understanding of empathy and support needs to recognize the full range of formal and informal support. It is interesting to note that the research procedures in themselves seem to have therapeutic benefits to the couples.

The last two chapters of this part focus on how gender influences the coping process and exchange of support within a relational context. Although both chapters also focus extensively on a particular stressor, chronic illness, the chapter by Acitelli and Badr builds on an interpersonal relationships framework and emphasizes the notion of relationship awareness; in contrast, the chapter by Revenson and her colleagues comes from a health psychology perspective and focuses on how the context of the illness shapes dyadic coping processes.

In chapter 6, Acitelli and Badr contend that how couples cope with chronic illness may depend on *who* is the ill spouse—the husband or wife. Whether spouses perceive the illness as *my* illness or *our* illness has implications for coping and the provision of support. They propose that it is better for the well-being of a relationship for partners to view the illness as a relationship issue rather than an individual issue. In support of this, they present findings from two studies that address the relationship between gender and relationship talk, with samples of "healthy" couples and couples coping with a serious illness. These data present a compelling case that men and women behave differently and expect different types of support from their partners depending on whether they are in the role of the patient or the well spouse. Furthermore, which spouse—the husband or the wife—engages in relationship talk will have an impact on the relationship satisfaction.

Revenson, Abraído-Lanza, Majerovitz, and Jordan expand on the influence of gender on dyadic coping in chapter 7 but use a social ecological model to guide their work. The conceptualization of coping congruence is used as a framework to analyze the *fit* between the partners' coping styles. To capture the interpersonal nature of coping, Revenson and her colleagues conducted a cluster analysis on coping behaviors of couples with rheumatic disease to describe how husbands and wives cope *as a unit* and how the medical, interpersonal, sociocultural, and temporal contexts affect couples' coping. The question, "What's gender got to do with it?" is addressed not only through these coping profiles but also by examining the division of household labor when either the husband or wife is ill.

The third and final part of this book focuses on specific psychosocial interventions with couples designed to enhance their coping with stress in general or with a specific stressor such as cancer. Widmer, Cina, Charvoz, Shantinath, and Bodenmann (chap. 8) describe their marital distress prevention program, Couples Coping Enhancement Training (CCET). This program integrates cognitive–behavioral approaches with theories of stress and coping and aims to strengthen the coping competencies of both partners through enhanced dyadic communication and dyadic coping. Based on the framework of dyadic coping presented in chapter 2, the six modules of the program focus on furthering partners' understanding and knowledge of stress, enhancing their individual coping and dyadic coping, improving their exchange and fairness in their relationships, fostering marital communication, and improving problem-solving skills. The authors present two outcome studies that evaluate the effectiveness of the program on marital quality, dyadic coping, individual coping, communication behaviors, and dyadic adjustment.

In chapter 9, Kayser describes an innovative couple-level intervention to assist couples who are coping with the recent diagnosis of breast cancer. The Partners in Coping Program (PICP) consists of a series of skill-based interventions designed to help couples enhance their interpersonal functioning (communication, coping strategies, problem solving, and emotional support), use help from others, realign family responsibilities, and provide continuity in their lives. This program is also based on the theory of dyadic stress and coping as conceptualized by Bodenmann (chap. 2) and employs cognitive–behavioral interventions with both partners. Preliminary findings from a clinical trial using a randomized group design support the intervention to enhance the dyadic coping of couples faced with the challenges of early-stage breast cancer.

The study of coping on a dyadic level represents a next step in understanding process as well as outcome, particularly when individuals are coping with stressors that affect both spouses. We cannot continue to separate the study of coping processes from that of social support. Whether we choose to conceptualize social support as a form of coping assistance (Thoits, 1986) or as a mode of coping (Bodenmann, 1997; O'Brien & DeLongis, 1997), much of what is considered coping involves the appraisals, actions, emotions, and feedback of others (Lazarus, 1999). Taken together, the chapters in this volume provide the field with both a new and exciting conceptualization of dyadic coping processes *and* a challenging set of unanswered questions that will guide future research.

References

Artis, J. E., & Pavalko, E. K. (2003). Explaining the decline in women's household labor: Individual change and cohort differences. *Journal of Marriage and Family, 65*, 746–761.

Bodenmann, G. (1995). A systemic-transactional view of stress and coping in couples. *Swiss Journal of Psychology, 54*, 34–49.

Bodenmann, G. (1997). Dyadic coping: A systemic-transactional view of stress and coping among couples: Theory and empirical findings. *European Review of Applied Psychology, 47*, 137–140.

Cohen, S., Kessler, R. C., & Gordon, L. U. (1997). *Measuring stress*. New York: Oxford University Press.

Coyne, J. C., & Fiske, V. (1992). Couples coping with chronic and catastrophic illness. In M. A. P. Stephens, S. E. Hobfoll, & J. Crowther (Eds.), *Family health psychology* (pp. 129–149). Washington, DC: Hemisphere Publication Services.

Crosby, F., & Jaskar, K. (1993). Women and men at home and at work: Realities and illusions. In S. Oskamp & M. Costanzo (Eds.), *Gender issues in social psychology* (pp. 143–171). Newbury Park, CA: Sage.

DeLongis, A., & O'Brien, T. B. (1990). An interpersonal framework for stress and coping: An application to the families of Alzheimer's patients. In M. A. P. Stephens, J. H. Crowther, S. E. Hobfoll, & D. L. Tennenbaum (Eds.), *Stress and coping in later-life families* (pp. 221–239). Washington, DC: Hemisphere Publication Services.

Kelly, J. G. (1971). The quest for valid preventive interventions. In G. Rosenblum (Ed.), *Issues in community psychology and preventive mental health* (pp. 109–139). New York: Behavioral Publications.

Lazarus, R. S. (1999). *Stress and emotion*. New York: Springer Publishing Company.

Lazarus, R. S., & Folkman, S. (1984). *Stress, appraisal and coping*. New York: Springer Publishing Company.

Lazarus, R. S., & Launier, R. (1978). Stress-related transactions between person and environment. In L. A. Pervin & M. Lewis (Eds.), *Perspectives in interactional psychology* (pp. 87–327). New York: Plenum Press.

Marks, N. F. (1996). Caregiving across the lifespan: National prevalence and predictors. *Family Relations, 45*, 27–36.

Marks, N. F., Lambert, J. D., & Choi, H. (2002). Transitions to caregiving, gender, and psychological well-being: A prospective U.S. national study. *Journal of Marriage and Family, 64*, 657–667.

O'Brien, T. B., & DeLongis, A. (1997). Coping with chronic stress: An interpersonal perspective. In B. Gottlieb (Ed.), *Coping with chronic stress* (pp. 161–190). New York: Plenum Press.

Pearlin, L. I., Lieberman, M., Menaghan, E., & Mullan, J. (1981). The stress process. *Journal of Health and Social Behavior, 22*, 337–356.

Pearlin, L. I., & Schooler, C. (1978). The structure of coping. *Journal of Health and Social Behavior, 19*, 2–21.

Putnam, R. D. (2000). *Bowling alone: The collapse and revival of American community*. New York: Simon & Schuster.

Revenson, T. A. (1994). Social support and marital coping with chronic illness. *Annals of Behavioral Medicine, 16*, 122–130.

Revenson, T. A. (2003). Scenes from a marriage: Examining support, coping, and gender within the context of chronic illness. In J. Suls & K. Wallston (Eds.), *Social psychological foundations of health and illness* (pp. 530–559). Oxford, England: Blackwell Publishing.

Schulz, R., O'Brien, T. B., Bookwala, J., & Fleissner, I. C. (1995). Psychiatric and physical morbidity effects of dementia caregiving: Prevalence, correlates and causes. *Gerontologist, 35*, 771–791.

Shelton, B. A., & John, D. (1996). The division of household labor. *Annual Review of Sociology, 22*, 299–322.

Thoits, P. A. (1986). Social support as coping assistance. *Journal of Consulting and Clinical Psychology, 54*, 416–423.

The Role of Stress in Dyadic Coping Processes

1

Marriages in Context: Interactions Between Chronic and Acute Stress Among Newlyweds

Benjamin R. Karney, Lisa B. Story, and Thomas N. Bradbury

In 1999, newspapers around the United States reported what many considered a startling finding. Census data collected the previous year revealed that Alabama, Arkansas, Oklahoma, and Tennessee had among the highest divorce rates in the country, around 50% higher than the national average. This was surprising because these four states constitute the heart of the Bible Belt, a region where conservative values and strong connection to religious organizations might have predicted lower divorce rates, not higher ones. Within those states and across the rest of the country, political leaders and policy makers were hard-pressed to explain the counterintuitive data.

Initial answers focused on expectations and education. For example, Jerry Reiger, Oklahoma's Secretary of Health and Human Services at the time, suggested to the press that "Kids don't have a very realistic view of marriage." To address this aspect of the problem, Oklahoma Governor Frank Keating initiated the Oklahoma Marriage Policy (Johnson et al., 2002), a collection of research and training programs designed to limit divorce and promote stable marriages. Arkansas Governor Mike Huckabee declared a "marital emergency" and promised immediate support for educational programs designed to lower his state's divorce rate. Other states soon followed suit. In Florida, lawmakers passed legislation offering engaged couples a discount on their marriage license if they can show evidence of taking a premarital education class. Marital education was also written into the high school curriculum, in the form of required classes teaching communication skills and relationship values. The theory underlying these efforts has rarely been made explicit, but it seems to be that high divorce rates are the result of a general misunderstanding of the chal-

Preparation of this article was supported by Grant MH59712 from the National Institute of Mental Health awarded to Benjamin R. Karney and by Grant MH48674 from the National Institute of Mental Health Awarded to Thomas N. Bradbury. This research was also supported in part by a grant to Benjamin R. Karney by the Fetzer Institute. Portions of this research were described at the 2001 meeting of the National Council on Family Relations in Rochester, NY.

We wish to thank Lisa Neff for her valuable insights and assistance with the preparation of this chapter.

lenges of marriage. Correcting this misunderstanding should therefore lower divorce rates and presumably lead to happier marriages.

The problem with this line of reasoning is that, on its face, a lack of education about marriage does not seem like a plausible explanation for the especially high divorce rates in the Bible Belt states. It might well be argued that there exists in the United States a romanticized view of marriage, but it would be hard to make the case that this view is more prevalent in the Bible Belt states than elsewhere. It may be reasonable to suggest that couples would benefit from improved communication skills, but it is difficult to find reasons why these skills would be especially lacking in the Bible Belt states compared to other parts of the country.

Explaining why Alabama, Arkansas, Oklahoma, and Tennessee have higher divorce rates than the other 46 states in the Union requires, as a first step, some effort to identify how these 4 states may differ from other states. To this end, the same data that revealed state-by-state disparities in divorce also point out other ways that these 4 states are distinct. According to the National Center for Health Statistics (National Center for Health Statistics, 2003), Alabama, Arkansas, Oklahoma, and Tennessee rank near the bottom of the 50 states in terms of employment rate, annual pay, household income, and health insurance coverage. At the same time, these states have among the highest rates of murder, infant mortality, and poverty in the nation. Whereas it is possible that couples in Alabama, Arkansas, Oklahoma, and Tennessee misunderstand the challenges of marriage, it is a certainty that life in general is more challenging in those states. The observation that divorce rates are higher in states where quality of life is poorer suggests an alternative explanation for the high divorce rates that lawmakers have yet to consider: Divorce and marital instability may sometimes result from challenges that are entirely external to spouses and their relationship. Marriages that survive and even thrive elsewhere may struggle in the face of unstable working conditions, neighborhoods beset by crime, poor education, and low wages.

The idea that external circumstances affect relationships may be counterintuitive to policy makers, but it is an old idea within research on couples and families. Some of the first theories to acknowledge the effects of stress on relationships were developed in the 1930s and 1940s when sociologists began to examine how families responded to the economic strains of the Great Depression and the military separations resulting from World War II. Hill's (1949) ABCX model of family stress made the links between the external and internal environment of a marriage explicit by suggesting that the stability of a family system was a product of the interaction between the stressful events experienced by families and the resources that families muster to cope with those events (for more recent elaborations, see Burr et al., 1994; McCubbin & Patterson, 1983).

In the last half century, empirical research on the effects of stress on families and relationships has generally lagged behind the pioneering theoretical developments of Hill and others, but a few propositions have been consistently supported. For example, the experience of a number of different stressors and stressful circumstances (e.g., receiving welfare, serving in the military, having a heart attack, and living in poverty) is on average associated with higher rates of marital dissolution (Bahr, 1979; Gimbel & Booth, 1994). Furthermore, the experience of stress external to the relationship has been specifically linked to more negative evaluations of the marriage (Bolger, DeLongis, Kessler, & Wethington, 1989; Tesser & Beach, 1998). There is even an emerging consensus that the quality of a couple's coping mediates the effects of stress on the relationship, such that stress exerts its negative effects by introducing opportunities for conflict and strain that would not otherwise be experienced by the couple (see chap. 2, this volume; Conger et al., 1990; Repetti, 1989). Accordingly, recent models of marriage and marital development assign the context in which the relationship develops a central role (Karney & Bradbury, 1995).

Despite this extensive literature, current understanding of the role of the external environment on relationships remains relatively unrefined. Although research and theory agree that, all else being equal, stress has adverse consequences for relationships, distinctions between kinds of stressful circumstances have yet to be explored systematically. Similarly, although stress is thought to predict poorer marital outcomes, research has yet to specify what kinds of negative outcomes are predicted by what kinds of stress. Finally, although there is an extensive literature debating the pros and cons of different approaches for measuring stress, there have been few attempts to demonstrate the empirical implications of different measurement strategies.

The goal of this chapter is to shed light on these issues, and in so doing, suggest directions for refining the current understanding of the effects of stressful circumstances on marriage. Toward this goal, the rest of the chapter is divided into three sections. First, we explore the possible implications of distinguishing among types of stress, dimensions of marital outcomes, and measurement strategies for specifying how marriages are affected by their context. Second, we summarize our recent empirical work addressing these issues through longitudinal data from newlywed couples. Finally, we discuss the broader implications of this work and identify further ways that models of stress and marriage may be elaborated.

The Context of Marriage: Life Events and Background Stressors

What does it mean to suggest that marriages are affected by their context? The context of a marriage can be defined as all of the actual and potential influences on a relationship that lie outside of the partners and their interaction. Thus, the context encompasses the daily challenges faced by each spouse, the major and minor life events they experience, enduring aspects of their socioeconomic status, and the cultural and historical milieu within which the relationship is embedded. Acknowledging the full breadth of the context of marriages points out the need for mapping the relevant elements of that context and identifying how those elements might interact. Yet, research to date has been slow to consider the context of a relationship as a whole. Instead, most research on how marriages and families are affected by their context has focused on single elements of the context at a time. For example, most studies examine associations between a specific life event (e.g., heart attack, death of a child, or military service), or a specific circumstance (e.g., low socioeconomic status or chronic unemployment), and marital outcomes.

The consistent results of such studies—more challenging events and circumstances are associated with poorer marital outcomes—might give the impression that different kinds of contextual factors affect marriages in basically the same way. However, these studies have generally overlooked potentially important dimensions on which elements of the context of a marriage may differ. For example, some aspects of the context are more proximal to the relationship than others (e.g., being in an automobile accident is more proximal than the historical milieu of the relationship). Some aspects of the context are more controllable than others (e.g., being fired is more controllable than experiencing a natural disaster). Some aspects of the context are current (e.g., being diagnosed with a serious illness), whereas others are historical (e.g., having recovered from a serious illness). Some aspects of the context directly affect both partners (e.g., the quality of the neighborhood), whereas some aspects directly affect only one partner (e.g., the quality of each partner's job). It seems likely that variability on each of these dimensions may moderate the effects of context on marriages, but to date those distinctions have been neither elaborated by theory nor addressed by empirical research.

Examining all of the dimensions of the context relevant to marriages is beyond the scope of this chapter. Rather, we focus here on one dimension that has been widely discussed and acknowledged, and yet seldom addressed in research on marriage and families—the distinction between chronic and acute stress. As commonly defined, chronic stresses or strains are those aspects of the context that are relatively stable and long lasting (e.g., socioeconomic status and having diabetes). These aspects of the context have also been referred to as background stressors (Gump & Matthews, 1999) because, although these aspects of the context represent constant drains on the resources of the relationship, they are unlikely to be salient in the daily lives of couples. In contrast, acute stressors are aspects of the context that have a specific onset and offset (e.g., a legal dispute or a transition between places of employment). Research on stressful life events has addressed acute stressors almost exclusively because the idea of an event implies an onset and an offset.

Prior research on chronic stressors (e.g., Bahr, 1979) and acute stressors (e.g., Cohan & Bradbury, 1997) indicate that both kinds of stressors are associated with negative marital outcomes. Yet careful consideration of the differences between the two kinds of stressors raises the possibility that each might give rise to those outcomes in distinct ways. For example, how should chronic stressors affect a marriage? Because chronic stressors are stable aspects of the environment, their effects should be enduring as well. Thus, couples experiencing chronically stressful conditions should experience more negative marital outcomes from the outset of the marriage. Furthermore, to the extent that chronic stressors create a constant drain on the resources of a couple, chronic stressors should inhibit a couple's efforts at relationship maintenance. Couples who must take several jobs to meet financial obligations, for example, are likely to have less time and energy to devote to romantic and exciting activities that may help to maintain satisfaction in less financially challenged relationships. Thus, we might expect that chronic stress should predict both relationship deterioration and poor relationship quality.

In contrast, how should acute events affect a marriage? Because acute stressors are, by definition, temporary, their effects may also be time limited. When a stressful life event occurs, partners' coping resources should be taxed, and their moods may be temporarily altered. Both of these things should affect the way partners experience and evaluate the relationship during that period. When the event ends, however, the possibility of a successful resolution of the stressor may free up previously committed coping resources. If the marriage is still deemed worth maintaining, those resources may be reallocated to relationship maintenance. Thus, it should be possible to recover from the negative effects of acute stress in a way that is less likely for chronic stress.

In addition to their distinct independent effects, chronic and acute stressors may also interact to affect marital outcomes. To the extent that experiencing an acute stressor presents an immediate challenge to the coping resources of a couple, then the experience of chronic stressor should affect the level of resources available to respond to that challenge. Couples who experience few chronic stresses may have high levels of resources to devote to coping with acute stressors. When such couples experience acute stress, coping may buffer the marriage from the effects of that stress. In contrast, couples who experience high levels of chronic stress should have fewer resources available when an acute stressor occurs. For these couples, the same acute stressor may present a more significant challenge to the relationship. In this way, levels of chronic stress might be expected to moderate the effects of acute stress on marital outcomes. Hill's (1949) original model of family stress proposed this sort of interaction, but although such interactions have indeed been demonstrated with respect to depression (Kuiper, Olinger, & Lyons, 1986) and physiological reactivity (Gump & Matthews, 1999), we are aware of no empirical research that has examined this interaction with respect to marital outcomes.

Can the experience of stress ever have positive effects on a relationship? Distinguishing between chronic and acute stressors suggests a possible answer to this question. The experience of an acute stressor may indeed be positive for couples whose levels of chronic stress are low and who have plenty of resources with which to cope with that stressor. For such couples, the experience of an acute stressor may be an opportunity to reinforce feelings of closeness and relational efficacy. Thus, accounting for the broader context of chronic stress in which acute stressors occur may affect not only the obtained magnitude of the effects of acute stress but the direction of those effects as well.

In sum, distinguishing between chronic and acute stressors suggests two ways that stress can affect marital outcomes. Acute or time-limited stressors should affect variability in marital outcomes, whereas chronic stressors should affect the overall course of the marriage, including reactions to acute stress. Given two couples, for example, one of whom faces financial uncertainty and one of whom is financially comfortable, the latter couple should have opportunities for romance that the former couple lacks. If both of these couples experience the same acute stressor, the couple already dealing with higher levels of chronic stress should have a harder time coping, and that should further affect the marriage negatively.

The Trajectory of Change in Marriage: Refining the Dependent Variable

When researchers examine the effects of external stress on marital outcomes, what marital outcomes are examined? The majority of research on these issues has examined just two dependent variables: the perceived quality of the relationship (i.e., marital satisfaction) and whether or not the marriage ends in divorce or permanent separation (i.e., marital dissolution). Both of these are static outcomes, drawing attention to the state of the marriage at a given time. Focusing on such outcomes may provide data on whether stress is generally associated with successful or unsuccessful marriages, but the prior discussion suggests that marriages can succeed or fail in different ways. Some marriages may be consistently satisfying or unsatisfying. Others may begin happily but then deteriorate. Distinguishing among these outcomes requires a more refined dependent variable than a single assessment can provide. Understanding the different ways that stress may affect marriage requires that researchers use longitudinal data to examine the full course of marriages over time.

Recent studies of newlywed marriage have adopted this approach, using multiple waves of data collected over several years to estimate individual trajectories of marital satisfaction for each spouse (Huston, Caughlin, Houts, Smith, & George, 2001; Karney & Bradbury, 1997). The trajectory can be estimated as a multifaceted dependent variable, with the number of parameters depending on the model of change used to describe each individual's data. The simplest linear model, for example, contains just two parameters: a level of satisfaction and a rate of change in satisfaction. Through multilevel modeling, each parameter of the trajectory can be examined simultaneously and independently (Bryk & Raudenbush, 1992). For example, the effects of stress on overall levels of marital satisfaction may be examined separately from the effects of stress on *change* in satisfaction over time. Similar approaches have been used to examine variability in relationship satisfaction, independent of levels of satisfaction or overall rates of change. Researchers drawing from extensive daily diary data have been able to examine how partners' feelings about their relationships covary with fluctuations in daily mood (Thompson & Bolger, 1999).

Understanding how marriages respond to different kinds of stressors may call for a combination of both these approaches. In the previous section, we raised the possibility that chronic stressors have independent effects on the overall quality of a relationship as well as spouses' ability to maintain the relationship. Testing this possibility suggests examining the effects of chronic stress on different parameters of the trajectory of spouses' satisfaction over time. Acute stress, in contrast, was described as having potentially time-varying effects. Testing this possibility suggests analyses that examine how fluctuations in acute stress and fluctuations in marital satisfaction covary across time. Such estimates require not only multiple waves of longitudinal data but also significant lengths of time. The potential benefit of such analyses is a richer picture of how marital outcomes may fluctuate as the demands of the context wax and wane.

Measuring Stress: Objective Versus Subjective Approaches

How do we know if a marriage is exposed to stress? One possibility is to obtain objective data about the environment of the marriage, such as demographic data or census data about specific neighborhoods. Relatively few studies have taken this approach (e.g., South, 2001). Instead, within the vast literature on stress, almost every answer to the question of measurement has involved some form of self-report. Given the difficulty of following individuals and observing the stressors to which they are exposed, the default option has been to rely on individuals' descriptions and recollections of their own stressful experiences. The strengths and limitations of this approach have been widely discussed (e.g., Cohen, Kessler, & Gordon, 1997), and this chapter is not the place to revisit that discussion. In an excellent summary of approaches to measuring stressful life events, Turner and Wheaton (1997) summarized much of the empirical literature and provided a list of recommendations for future researchers interested in studying stressful events specifically. Focusing on checklist methods of assessing stressful events, they recommend tailoring the list of events to the populations being studied and excluding events that are clearly positive (positive experiences showing few important consequences in previous literature). The number of negative events experienced during a given period can be a rough indicator of the amount of acute stress an individual has had to cope with during that period.

Yet even these recommendations leave researchers with several options for determining which events are negative and which are positive. Different approaches vary in the extent to which they take the subjective experience of the individual into account. For example, some measures allow respondents to decide which events are negative by asking them to rate the impact of each event they endorse from a given list. The sum of all of the events that the individual rates as negative represents their experience of acute stress. This approach has some face validity, but it is limited in that different people given the same list of events might differ in their evaluation of those events as positive or negative. The danger is that unmeasured individual differences (e.g., neuroticism) might lead some individuals to rate as negative some events that are not negative for most people. For these individuals, the number of events they endorse would confound their experiences with their stable perceptual biases. A more conservative approach would be to determine the positivity or negativity of each event on the basis of sample-wide data. The advantage of this approach is that a sum of negative events represents the experience of events that most people agree are negative, independent of the perceptual tendencies of the respondent. On the other hand, such an index might also lead to confusing results, as the sum of negative events for an individual could include events that the individual actually perceived as nonstressful or positive.

In the absence of a literature that resolves the question, the best approach might be to evaluate acute stress both ways and determine whether the difference in measurement strategy affects results. In research on a dependent variable that is inherently subjective, such as marital satisfaction, we might expect that the more conservative approach, removing an element of subjectivity from the acute stress scores, would reveal fewer significant effects than an approach that takes the subjective experience of the individual into account.

A Longitudinal Study of Stress and Marital Satisfaction in Newlyweds

Elaborating on existing models of stress and marriage highlights the potential value in making distinctions that previous research in this area has overlooked. Chronic and acute stressors are likely to have unique and even interactive effects on marital outcomes. Levels of satisfaction in a marriage may be affected differently than rates of change or variability in marital satisfaction over time. Examining events that the individual perceives to be stressful may provide a different picture than examining events that are judged to be stressful by others.

In this section, we summarize our recent research that addresses these distinctions (Karney, Story, & Bradbury, 2004). In the study described here, a sample of first-married newlyweds provided data on their marital satisfaction and their experiences of chronic and acute stress every 6 months for the first 4 years of their marriages. Growth curve modeling allowed us to address three specific questions. First, do self-reports of chronic stress and self-reports of acute stress affect different parameters of the trajectory of marital satisfaction? Second, do levels of chronic stress moderate the covariance between fluctuations in acute stress and variability in marital satisfaction? Finally, do the obtained associations among these variables differ depending on whether stressful life events are measured subjectively or objectively?

Methods of Studying Stress and Marriage

Our approach to addressing these questions has been to solicit newlywed couples through their marriage licenses applications. Why newlyweds? Examining newly married couples provides several advantages in research on stress and relationship development. First, compared to more established marriages, newly married couples experience more dramatic changes in relationship quality and are at elevated risk of marital disruption (Cherlin, 1992). Newlyweds are thus an appropriate sample in which to examine issues of change and stability. Second, couples in the early years of marriage are likely to be exposed to a wide variety of stressful life events, as a number of stressors tend to accompany the transition to marriage (e.g., relocation and starting a new job). In the later years of marriage, more stable circumstances and the likelihood of children may reduce the role of external stress in couples' lives as the strains within the family itself increase.

Couples eligible on the basis of information available on their licenses are typically sent letters inviting them to participate in a longitudinal study of marriage. Interested couples are screened further for eligibility with a telephone interview to determine that this is the first marriage for both spouses; the couple has been married less than 6 months; neither partner has children;

both partners are over 18 years old and wives are less than 35 years old (so that couples might become parents over the course of the study); both spouses speak English and have received at least a 10th-grade education; and the couple has no immediate plans to move away from the area.

The sample described in this chapter comprised 172 couples who met the eligibility criteria and kept their first laboratory appointment. Over 60% of husbands and wives were Caucasian, and at the time of initial data collection, all couples had been married less than 6 months. (For more details about this sample, see Karney & Frye, 2002)

Couples were mailed a packet of questionnaires to complete at home and then were scheduled to attend a 3-hour laboratory session during which spouses completed additional questionnaires, were interviewed individually, and participated in dyadic interaction tasks. At approximately 6-month intervals, couples were mailed additional packets of questionnaires to complete at home. The third follow-up also included an in-person laboratory session, but for all other follow-ups, spouses returned their questionnaires by mail. By the end of the study, we had gathered eight waves of data, covering approximately the first 4 years of marriage.

Although a number of couples divorced over the course of the study, retention was relatively high. At the eighth wave of data collection, approximately 4 years after the initial assessment, marital status was known for 100% of the original 172 couples. Of those couples, 13 (8%) had experienced divorce or permanent separation. Among intact couples, 62% of husbands and 65% of wives provided data at Time 8. Independent-sample t tests revealed that spouses who provided data at Time 8 did not differ from spouses who failed to provide data on any of the variables examined in this chapter (all $ts < 1.6$). One of the advantages of the strategy used to analyze these data is that participants who did not provide data at every time point could be included in all analyses. In this study, 157 (91%) of the original 172 couples were retained in the analyses.

MEASURING MARITAL SATISFACTION. To ensure that perceptions of stress and evaluations of the marriage were not confounded (Fincham & Bradbury, 1987; Huston, McHale, & Crouter, 1986), marital satisfaction was measured using an instrument that assessed global sentiments toward the marriage exclusively. At every assessment, spouses completed a version of the Semantic Differential (SMD; Osgood, Suci, & Tannenbaum, 1957), an instrument that asks participants to rate their perception of the marriage on 7-point scales between two opposite adjectives. In the current study, spouses rated how they felt about their marriage on 15 adjective pairs (e.g., *bad–good*, *dissatisfied–satisfied*, and *unpleasant–pleasant*). The internal consistency of this measure was high (across waves of measurement, coefficient alpha averaged above .95 for both spouses).

MEASURING ACUTE STRESS. To assess spouses' experiences of acute stress during each 6-month interval, couples completed at each assessment a version of the Life Experiences Survey (LES; Sarason, Johnson, & Siegel, 1978). This version of the LES presented spouses with a list of 192 events that had been selected from other standardized life events checklists to emphasize acute stressors likely to occur in a young, married population. For each event, spouses were first asked to indicate whether the event had occurred over the preceding 6 months (i.e., since the last wave of assessment). If the event had occurred, spouses were then asked to indicate the impact the event had on their lives on a 7-point scale ranging from extremely negative (−3) to extremely positive (+3). Each stressful event then had to meet two criteria to be included in the final composite score. First, the event could not represent a likely consequence of marital satisfaction, marital distress, or depression. Nineteen items (e.g., emotional difficulties, major change in sleeping habits, and relationship with spouse worsened a lot) were excluded from the final score for this reason. In this way, the measure was designed to tap only those stressors external to (i.e., unlikely to be a consequence of) the conditions of the marriage. Second, consistent with the recommendations of Turner and Wheaton (1997), the event had to represent a negative life stressor.

Two different approaches were used to compute final acute stress scores at each assessment. First, we computed a sum for each spouse that excluded all of the events that the spouse indicated were positive. Within this approach, the acute stress score accounted for the subjective evaluation of the individual and represented the number of life events that each individual perceived to be negative during the 6 months. Second, we used the data from the entire sample to determine which events were considered to be positive or negative on a sample-wide basis. Events that were on average rated by the sample as positive during a majority of time points were excluded from the final list of events. Within this approach, the acute stress score was less subjective and represented the number of events from the remaining list that each spouse reported experiencing during the 6 months. In describing the results below, we begin by reporting results from the first approach and then describe how the pattern of results changed after we adopted the second, more stringent approach.

MEASURING CHRONIC STRESS. During their initial laboratory visit at Time 1, each spouse was interviewed individually to assess chronic stress using a modification of a protocol developed by Hammen et al. (1987). Spouses were asked to describe in detail the quality of the following nine life domains over the prior 6 months: the marital relationship, relationships with family, relationships with in-laws, relationships with friends, experiences at school, experiences at work, finances, own health, and spouse's health. For each domain, interviewers were instructed to probe for concrete indicators of the ongoing stressors that the spouse may be experiencing. After describing each domain, spouses were instructed to rate their experiences within that domain over the prior 6 months on a 9-point scale, where a *1* indicated exceptionally positive circumstances and a *9* indicated exceptionally stressful circumstances. At Time 3, when spouses returned to the laboratory for a second interview, the same procedure was used to assess chronic stress. At all other follow-up assessments, spouses read through a series of questions about each domain (taken from the initial interview) and then were asked to rate their experiences in the same way as during their interviews. Because the current analyses were not concerned with chronic stress in any specific domain, ratings from the eight nonmarital domains of the interview were averaged at each assessment to form a score indicating the overall level of nonmarital chronic stress experienced by each spouse during each 6-month interval.

To assess the validity of spouses' self-ratings of chronic stress, the interviewers were also asked to make ratings of the chronic stress experienced by spouses in each domain using the same scales that the spouses used. Interviewers' mean ratings of chronic stress were significantly correlated with husbands' and wives' ratings of their own stress at Time 1 (for husbands, $r = .54$, $p < .01$; for wives, $r = .65$, $p < .01$) and Time 3 (for husbands, $r = .51$, $p < .01$; for wives, $r = .64$, $p < .01$). Thus, spouses' self-reports of their chronic stress at each assessment appeared to represent a reasonable assessment of their actual experiences.

DATA ANALYSIS. As in much of our longitudinal research, the central analyses of this study were conducted with hierarchical linear modeling (HLM; Bryk & Raudenbush, 1992) and the HLM/2L computer program (Bryk, Raudenbush, & Congdon, 1994). This approach to the analysis of multiwave longitudinal data typically proceeds in two stages. First, multiple assessments of a variable are used to estimate a trajectory, or growth curve, to describe how that variable changes over time for each individual in a sample. Second, the parameters summarizing the change of each individual are treated as new dependent measures, allowing researchers to examine whether individual deviations from the average trajectory are associated with other within-subject or between-subjects variables.

The HLM approach has several advantages over other available approaches to analyzing trajectories (e.g., structural equation modeling). First, HLM provides reliable estimates of within-subject parameters of change even when sample sizes are relatively small. Second, HLM uses all available data from each individual to estimate within-subject parameters. Thus, participants who do not have data at every time point could be included in the analyses. Third, HLM computes effects on each parameter through simultaneous equations; thus effects on one parameter of change are estimated controlling for effects on other parameters of change. Finally, HLM allows for husbands' and wives' trajectories to be estimated simultaneously in a couple-level model (e.g., Raudenbush, Brennan, & Barnett, 1995), thereby controlling for dependencies in husbands' and wives' data.

What Do Longitudinal Assessments of Chronic and Acute Stress Look Like?

Mean chronic stress, acute stress, and marital satisfaction scores at each assessment are described in Table 1.1. Mean marital satisfaction scores at each assessment declined over time. Indeed, prior analyses of this sample (Davila, Karney, Hall, & Bradbury, 2003; Karney & Frye, 2002) have demonstrated that for both spouses marital satisfaction becomes on average significantly less positive and more variable over the first 4 years of marriage. With respect to acute stress, both spouses' reports declined over the first 2 years of marriage and then remained relatively stable over the second 2 years.

Table 1.1. Descriptive Statistics for Husbands and Wives

Partner	Assessment time							
	1	2	3	4	5	6	7	8
Marital satisfaction								
Husband								
M	94.7	92.1	94.0	92.3	91.9	92.0	89.8	90.8
SD	9.6	12.5	11.0	12.6	14.3	13.5	15.6	15.1
Wife								
M	97.2	94.7	96.0	94.5	92.9	91.0	91.2	90.3
SD	8.4	12.2	11.8	12.2	15.5	17.1	16.8	16.6
Acute stress								
Husband								
M	7.4	6.3	5.7	4.7	5.0	4.8	4.1	4.9
SD	5.1	5.6	5.0	4.2	4.5	4.4	3.8	4.8
Wife								
M	9.5	7.3	5.6	5.6	6.2	5.3	4.5	5.3
SD	6.2	5.51	4.6	4.6	5.6	5.3	4.3	4.4
Chronic stress								
Husband								
M	2.8	3.1	2.9	3.0	3.1	3.1	3.0	3.1
SD	.7	.8	.7	.7	.8	.8	.8	.9
Wife								
M	2.9	3.0	2.9	3.0	3.1	3.0	3.1	3.2
SD	.6	.7	.7	.7	.8	.7	.8	.8

Note. The pattern of means and standard deviations remained the same when only those couples who presented data at every time point were included (n = 64). Each time point is separated by a period of 6 months with Time 1 occurring within in the first 6 months of marriage.

Repeated-measures ANOVAs with linear contrasts confirmed that the overall decline was significant for husbands, $F(1,71) = 26.4$, $p < .001$, effect-size $r = .52$, and for wives, $F(1,75) = 57.7$, $p < .001$, effect-size $r = .66$. With respect to chronic stress, both spouses' reports increased slightly over time. This pattern was significant for wives, $F(1, 75) = 17.2$, $p < .001$, effect-size $r = .43$, but not for husbands, $F(1, 71) = 2.3$, $p = .14$, effect-size $r = .18$. Across the eight waves of assessment, the mean standard deviation of spouses' acute stress scores was 5.7 for husbands and 6.5 for wives. The mean standard deviation for chronic stress scores was 3.5 for husbands and 3.8 for wives. Although reports of both kinds of stress demonstrated some mean change over time, reports of chronic stress were, as expected, more stable (i.e., more chronic) than were reports of acute stress.

As a preliminary test of the associations among these measures, within-spouse correlations among the measures were examined at each time point. Consistent with prior research by Pearlin and colleagues (e.g., Pearlin, Mullan, Semple, & Skaff, 1990; Pearlin & Turner, 1995), reports of chronic and acute stress were significantly associated for both spouses (across assessments, rs ranged from .22 to .48 for husbands and from .29 to .52 for wives), such that spouses who reported higher levels of chronic stress also reported higher levels of acute stress. Chronic stress scores were significantly associated with marital satisfaction at 7 of the 8 assessments for husbands (rs ranged from −.11 to −.38 across assessments) and at 6 of the 8 assessments for wives (rs ranged from −.11 to −.39 across assessments), such that higher chronic stress was associated with lower marital satisfaction. Acute stress was associated with marital satisfaction to a lesser degree at 4 of the 8 assessments for husbands (rs ranged from −.02 to −.35 across assessments) and 6 of the 8 assessments for wives (rs ranged from −.50 to .03 across assessments), such that spouses who were experiencing higher acute stress reported lower marital satisfaction.

Correlations between husbands' and wives' reports of marital satisfaction were significant at every assessment (across spouses and assessments, rs ranged from .36 to .66), offering support for the idea that spouses were responding to their shared relationship. Spouses' reports of acute stress were significantly associated in 6 out of the 8 assessments (between-spouse rs ranged from .09 to .39), and their reports of chronic stress were significantly associated at 7 out of 8 assessments (rs ranged from .04 to .37).

In sum, preliminary analyses confirmed that mean acute stress and chronic stress scores change over time. Whereas acute stress decreased, chronic stress increased over time. However, there was substantial individual variability in reported stress among these spouses (see Table 1.1). Determining whether the variability in acute stress generalized to the individual level required that both measures be submitted to a growth curve analysis.

ANALYZING CHANGE IN ACUTE STRESS. Prior analyses of this data set (e.g., Karney & Frye, 2002) found that change in satisfaction over the first 4 years of marriage could be best described by a linear function, summarizing the repeated marital satisfaction scores of each spouse in terms of an initial level (an intercept) and a rate of linear change over time (a slope). To date, we are aware of no longitudinal research examining the appropriateness of different models of change in acute stress. To determine the models that best describe how spouses' self-reports of acute stress change over the first years of marriage, we compared two different models as descriptions of the repeated assessments.

The first was a mean and variance model, suggesting that levels of acute stress do not develop systematically over time but rather vary randomly at each assessment around an individual's mean level. To evaluate this model, the following function was specified to describe the data from each individual:

$$Y_{ij} = B_{oj} + r_{ij} \tag{1}$$

where Y_{ij} is the stress score of individual j at Time i; B_{oj} is the mean level of stress of individual j across assessments; and r_{ij} is the deviation from the mean level at each assessment. This model provided reliable estimates of husbands' and wives' mean levels of acute stress (.84 for husbands and .88 for wives).

The alternative model was a linear model, which allows for the possibility that acute stress does not vary randomly between intervals but rather develops systematically over the first years of marriage. This model can be described by the following function:

$$Y_{ij} = B_{oj} + B_{1j}(\text{time}) + r_{ij} \tag{2}$$

where the slope term, B_{1j}, represents the rate of change in attribution scores over time. Estimating this model produced reliable estimates for husbands and wives of the intercepts (.81 for husbands and .79 for wives) and of slopes (.66 for husbands and .64 for wives). For both spouses, the mean estimated slopes differed significantly from 0, for husbands, $t(156) = -5.9$, $p < .001$, and for wives, $t(156) = -7.4$, p < .001. Because the first model is nested within the second, the difference between their goodness of fit statistics can be tested as a chi-square to compare the appropriateness of the two models. For both spouses, the difference between the models was significant ($X^2 = 260.6$, $df = 2$, $p < .05$ for husbands and $X^2 = 301.4$, $df = 2$, $p < .05$ for wives), suggesting that the linear change model described the data better than the simpler mean and variance model. Given that acute stress appears to decline over time in this sample, acute stress was treated as a time-varying covariate of marital satisfaction in all subsequent analyses.

How Does Acute Stress Affect the Trajectory of Marital Satisfaction?

To examine the effects of variability in spouses' levels of acute stress on the development of their marital satisfaction, acute stress scores were centered around the mean level for each spouse and then entered into the model summarizing the trajectory of marital satisfaction for each spouse. Thus, the development of each spouse's satisfaction was modeled with the following equation:

$$Y_{ij} = B_{0j} + B_{1j}(\text{time}) + B_{2j}(\text{acute stress}) + r_{ij} \tag{3}$$

where Y_{ij} represents the satisfaction of Spouse i at Time j, B_{0j} represents the intercept, or the initial level of satisfaction for Spouse i, B_{1j} represents the slope, or the rate of linear change in satisfaction over time for Spouse i, B_{2j} represents the covariance between changes in satisfaction and changes in acute stress for Spouse i, controlling for the overall trajectory of satisfaction for that spouse, and r_{ij} represents error, assumed to be independent and normally distributed across spouses. Within this model, a significant estimate of B_{2j} would indicate that changes in a spouse's reports of acute stress between intervals tend to be associated with corresponding changes in a spouse's marital satisfaction, controlling for the overall rate of change in marital satisfaction for that spouse.

Once the parameters of Equation 3 were estimated for each spouse, the crucial statistic was the mean of the coefficient for acute stress, the time-varying covariate B_{2j}. This coefficient was significant and negative for husbands and for wives: for husbands, beta = $-.25$, $t(156) = -4.2$, $p < .001$, effect-size $r = -.30$; for wives, beta = $-.15$, $t(156) = -2.0$, $p < .05$, effect-size $r = -.14$. The significant coefficients confirm that variability in acute stress accounted for significant variability in the trajectory for both spouses. Controlling for their overall rates of change over time, we found that spouses tended to report lower marital satisfaction when their reports of acute stress were higher than average and higher marital satisfaction when their reports of acute stress were lower than average.

How Does Chronic Stress Affect the Trajectory of Marital Satisfaction?

Relative to their reports of acute stress, spouses' reports of chronic stress were comparatively stable. The repeated assessments of chronic stress were averaged to form a mean chronic stress score for each spouse, representing the average level of chronic stress reported by each spouse across the first 4 years of marriage. These scores were then used to account for between-spouse variability in the parameters of the within-spouse model described in Equation 3. Because these analyses estimate associations between chronic stress and each parameter of the within-spouse model simultaneously, these analyses provide the unique associations between chronic stress and each parameter of the trajectory of marital satisfaction, controlling for the associations between chronic stress and each of the other parameters of the within-spouse model. The results of these analyses are reported in Table 1.2.

As Table 1.2 indicates, chronic stress scores were uniquely associated with each parameter of the trajectory of marital satisfaction. With respect to the intercepts, this association was significant and negative for both spouses regardless of the measure used to assess the trajectory. Consistent with our expectations, spouses who reported higher levels of chronic stress across the first 4 years of marriage reported lower levels of marital satisfaction at the beginning of the marriage and at every assessment thereafter. With respect to the slopes, the association was again in the expected direction and significant for both spouses. Controlling for the effects of chronic stress on initial levels of satisfaction, we found higher levels of chronic stress were associated with steeper declines in marital satisfaction over time.

Table 1.2. Effects of Chronic Stress on the Trajectory of Satisfaction and Acute Stress

Partner	Coefficient	SE	t	Effect-size r
	Effects on intercepts			
Husband	−2.9	1.3	−2.3*	−.17
Wife	−3.1	1.3	−2.4*	−.17
	Effects on slopes			
Husband	−0.6	.2	−2.6*	−.20
Wife	−0.9	.3	−3.3**	−.25
	Effects on within-subject covariation with acute stress			
Husband	−.14	.1	−1.4	−.11
Wife	−.20	.1	−2.0*	−.15

Note. $n = 157$ husbands and 157 wives.
*$p < .05$, **$p < .01$, ***$p < .001$.

DO CHRONIC AND ACUTE STRESSORS INTERACT? Of central interest to the current analyses was the association between chronic stress and the coefficient of the time-varying covariate. This is the association that addresses the moderation hypothesis: Do levels of chronic stress moderate the within-subject association between marital satisfaction and acute stress? This effect was significant for wives only (see Table 1.2). For wives experiencing higher levels of chronic stress, marital satisfaction was significantly more reactive to changes in acute stress; whereas for wives experiencing lower levels of chronic stress, marital satisfaction was less reactive to changes in acute stress.

To what extent did chronic stress account for the association between fluctuations in acute stress and variability in marital satisfaction? To address this question, we examined the same coefficients described earlier (i.e., the within-subject association between changes in acute stress and changes in marital satisfaction) after between-subjects differences in chronic stress were controlled. Once chronic stress was controlled, the negative associations between acute stress and marital satisfaction were no longer significant. In fact, the association was positive for both spouses and nearly significantly so for wives: for husbands, beta = .21, $t(156)$ = .71, ns, effect-size r = .03; for wives, beta = .48, $t(156)$ = 1.65, $p < .10$, effect-size r = −.13. In other words, absent chronic stress, there is a trend toward satisfaction covarying positively with acute stress. For couples who have the coping resources, marital satisfaction may grow during periods when acute stress is higher than average.

DOES A MORE STRINGENT MEASURE OF ACUTE STRESS CHANGE THE RESULTS? Thus far, all of the results involving acute stress have examined an index that summed the number of events that each spouse rated as negative. Such a measure introduces an element of subjectivity to the acute stress index, as different spouses may have evaluated the positivity or negativity of each event differently. How did these results change when a more stringent measure of acute stress was used, one that determined the valence of each event using data from the entire sample rather than the individual? As expected, minimizing the subjective experience of the spouse weakened all of the results involving acute stress. For husbands, the pattern of significant results did not change. That is, fluctuations in the more objective acute stress measure continued to covary significantly with variability in marital satisfaction, though the effect size was reduced from −.30 to −.22. Husbands' chronic stress still failed to moderate this association. For wives, the within-subject association between acute stress and marital satisfaction was reduced to nonsignificance (the effect size weakened from −.14 to −.05), leaving no effect for chronic stress to moderate.

Making Sense of the Effects of Stress on Marriage

A marriage exists within a rich context that includes the experiences of each spouse outside of the relationship and ranges to include the stable quality of their environment and the historical era in which they live. Yet, to date, the complexity of the potential contextual influences on marriage has not been reflected in research. Instead, studies of how marriages may be affected by external stress have tended to address single elements of the context, focusing on a specific life event (e.g., a heart attack) or a particular aspect of the social context (e.g., a high crime rate). A similar lack of differentiation has characterized the assessment of marital outcomes. Although marriage is an inherently temporal phenomenon, unfolding and developing through time, researchers have tended to emphasize static marital outcomes, such as divorce or marital satisfaction, at a single assessment. The study summarized in this chapter (Karney et al., 2004) sheds light on the complexity that research in this area has often overlooked in hopes of contributing to more refined models of stress and coping in marriage.

We suggested that chronic stressors, representing stable aspects of the environment, should represent a constant drain on the resources of a couple. Thus, we expected that higher levels of chronic stressors would be associated with lower levels of satisfaction as well as satisfaction that declined more steeply over time. Indeed, spouses who reported higher average levels of chronic stress during the first years of marriage reported lower marital satisfaction at the outset of the marriage and at every assessment thereafter. Furthermore, controlling for this effect, we found that spouses who reported higher average levels of chronic stress also experienced satisfaction that deteriorated more quickly over time. It seems that it is harder to maintain even moderate levels of satisfaction when the context of the marriage makes constant demands on a couple's resources.

Acute stress appeared to have very different effects on the trajectory of marital satisfaction. By definition, levels of acute stress fluctuate over time. Thus, we expected that the effects of acute stress on marital satisfaction would also be time limited. In fact, marital satisfaction did covary with fluctuations in acute stress over time. Controlling for overall declines in marital satisfaction, we found that satisfaction was especially high when levels of acute stress were relatively low and especially low during periods when acute stress was relatively high. Most significantly, the magnitude of this association appeared to depend on the stable level of chronic stress to which the marriage was exposed. At least for wives, the negative association between acute stress and marital satisfaction was strongest when levels of chronic stress were relatively high. In other words, when the external context contains constant drains on a couple's coping resources, the experience of acute negative events has an especially negative effect on wives' marital satisfaction. It is not hard to imagine examples that illustrate this idea. If one member of a couple is injured in an automobile accident, clearly the effect that this event has on the rest of their lives together will depend at least in part on stable qualities of their lives, such as whether they have a second car or whether they have adequate health insurance. If a couple lacks resources to cope with the negative events they encounter, it makes sense that those events will be especially consequential.

When a couple does possess adequate resources, however, the experience of a negative event external to the relationship may be positive, an opportunity for spouses to support each other and thereby come closer together. Results from this study provide tentative support for this idea. When levels of chronic stress were statistically controlled (i.e., extrapolating from these data to a point at which chronic stress is zero), the association between fluctuations in acute stress and variability in marital satisfaction was no longer significant for either spouse. In fact, the association was flipped in the positive direction for both spouses. In other words, when a couple possesses adequate resources to cope successfully with the negative events they experience, surmounting the challenge those events represent may leave couples closer than before.

In addressing these associations, we also compared two approaches to measuring negative life events. One approach created an index of negative events from the events that each spouse, perhaps idiosyncratically, rated as negative. The other created the index from the list of events determined to be negative for most people through analyses of sample-wide ratings of each event. As expected, results using the second, more objective method were weaker. For wives in particular, the interaction between chronic and acute stress was only obtained using the less objective measure. Why might this be so? One possibility is that for wives in this study, the subjective experience of acute stress may affect evaluations of the marriage more than the objective nature of the stressors.

Different kinds of stress accounted for relatively small amounts of variance in the trajectory of marital satisfaction, even when the associations were significant. It is worth noting, however, that the sample represented a very narrow range of stress. For the most part, this sample consisted of young, middle-class, well-educated couples. The sample did not include couples at the ends of the stress continuum, those likely to possess vast resources and those likely to face the most severe chronic stressors. Thus, the analyses described here provided a highly conservative test of these ideas. In a general population encompassing the full range of chronic stress and levels of resources, more variance in marital outcome might be accounted for. If these data are any indication, then the overall quality of people's lives should play a substantial role in the development of their relationships. When life is good, marriages should be happier, easier to maintain, and less reactive to negative events. When life is bad, marriages should be less happy, harder to maintain, and more vulnerable to acute stress. Further support for these ideas would emphasize that understanding marital processes requires that the context within which those processes are occurring be taken into account.

Conclusion

So, what can be done about the especially high divorce rates in Alabama, Arkansas, Oklahoma, and Tennessee? The solutions currently being pursued—skills training and education about relationships—may be a valuable beginning, but they imply that the only determinants of marital outcomes are the two members of a couple and the nature of the interaction between them. The data summarized here, although they did not directly address state-by-state comparisons, nevertheless offer a different view. One reason marriages may be failing in the states of the Bible Belt is that life is hard in those states. Facing high crime, high unemployment, and little access to health insurance—all chronic stressors—couples may lack resources they might otherwise devote to maintaining and enhancing their relationships. Under these conditions, marriages may begin less happy, deteriorate more rapidly, and finally dissolve in the face of acute negative life events. If replicated in a broader population, such findings would suggest radically different strategies for reducing the pain and cost associated with divorce. Rather than developing programs targeted specifically at relationships, policy makers might consider supporting programs aimed at raising standards of living. When provided with an external context that supports the relationship, couples may be well equipped to maintain their relationships on their own.

References

Bahr, S. J. (1979). The effects of welfare on marital stability and remarriage. *Journal of Marriage and the Family, 41*, 553–560.

Bolger, N., DeLongis, A., Kessler, R. C., & Wethington, E. (1989). The contagion of stress across multiple roles. *Journal of Marriage and the Family, 51*, 175–183.

Bryk, A. S., & Raudenbush, S. W. (1992). *Hierarchical linear models: Applications and data analysis methods*. Newbury Park, CA: Sage.

Bryk, A. S., Raudenbush, S. W., & Congdon, R. T. (1994). *HLM: Hierarchical linear modelling with the HLM/2L and HLM/3L programs*. Chicago: Scientific Software International.

Burr, W. R., Klein, S., Burr, R. G., Doxey, C., Harker, B., Holman, T. B., et al. (1994). *Reexamining family stress: New theory and research* (Vol. 193). Thousand Oaks, CA: Sage.

Cherlin, A. J. (1992). *Marriage, divorce, remarriage* (2nd ed.). Cambridge, MA: Harvard University Press.

Cohan, C. L., & Bradbury, T. N. (1997). Negative life events, marital interaction, and the longitudinal course of newlywed marriage. *Journal of Personality and Social Psychology, 73*, 114–128.

Cohen, S., Kessler, R. C., & Gordon, L. U. (1997). *Measuring stress: A guide for health and social scientists*. New York: Oxford University Press.

Conger, R. D., Elder, G. H., Lorenz, F. O., Conger, K. J., Simons, R. L., Whitbeck, L. B., et al. (1990). Linking economic hardship to marital quality and instability. *Journal of Marriage and the Family, 52*, 643–656.

Davila, J., Karney, B. R., Hall, T. W., & Bradbury, T. N. (2003). Depressive symptoms and marital satisfaction: Dynamic associations and the moderating effects of gender and neuroticism. *Journal of Family Psychology, 17*, 557–570.

Fincham, F. D., & Bradbury, T. N. (1987). The assessment of marital quality: A reevaluation. *Journal of Marriage and the Family, 49*, 797–809.

Gimbel, C., & Booth, A. (1994). Why does military combat experience adversely affect marital relations? *Journal of Marriage and the Family, 56*, 691–703.

Gump, B. B., & Matthews, K. A. (1999). Do background stressors influence reactivity to and recovery from acute stressors? *Journal of Applied Social Psychology, 29*, 469–494.

Hammen, C., Adrien, C., Gordon, D., Burge, D., Jaenicke, C., & Hiroto, D. (1987). Children of depressed mothers: Maternal strain and symptom predictors of dysfunction. *Journal of Abnormal Psychology, 96*, 190–198.

Hill, R. (1949). *Families under stress*. New York: Harper & Row.

Huston, T. L., Caughlin, J. P., Houts, R. M., Smith, S. E., & George, L. J. (2001). The connubial crucible: Newlywed years as predictors of marital delight, distress, and divorce. *Journal of Personality and Social Psychology, 80*, 237–254.

Huston, T. L., McHale, S. M., & Crouter, A. C. (1986). When the honeymoon's over: Changes in the marriage relationship over the first year. In R. Gilmore & S. Duck (Eds.), *The emerging field of personal relationships* (pp. 109–132). Hillsdale, NJ: Erlbaum.

Johnson, C. A., Stanley, S. M., Glenn, N. D., Amato, P. R., Nock, S. L., Markman, H. J., & Dion, M. R. (2002). *Marriage in Oklahoma: 2001 baseline statewide survey on marriage and divorce*. Oklahoma City: Bureau for Social Research, Oklahoma State University.

Karney, B. R., & Bradbury, T. N. (1995). The longitudinal course of marital quality and stability: A review of theory, method, and research. *Psychological Bulletin, 118*, 3–34.

Karney, B. R., & Bradbury, T. N. (1997). Neuroticism, marital interaction, and the trajectory of marital satisfaction. *Journal of Personality and Social Psychology, 72*, 1075–1092.

Karney, B. R., & Frye, N. E. (2002). "But we've been getting better lately": Comparing prospective and retrospective views of relationship development. *Journal of Personality and Social Psychology, 82,* 222–238.

Karney, B. R., Story, L. B., & Bradbury, T. N. (2004). *Interactions between chronic and acute stress in newlywed marriage.* Manuscript in preparation.

Kuiper, N. A., Olinger, L. J., & Lyons, L. M. (1986). Global perceived stress level as a moderator of the relationship between negative life events and depression. *Journal of Human Stress, 12*(4), 149–153.

McCubbin, H. I., & Patterson, J. M. (1983). Family transitions: Adaptation to stress. In H. I. McCubbin & C. R. Figley (Eds.), *Stress and the family: Coping with normative transitions* (Vol. 1, pp. 5–25). New York: Brunner/Mazel.

National Center for Health Statistics. (2003, July 14). Retrieved July 16, 2003, from http://www.cdc.gov/nchs/

Osgood, C. E., Suci, G. J., & Tannenbaum, P. H. (1957). *The measurement of meaning.* Urbana: University of Illinois Press.

Pearlin, L. I., Mullan, J. T., Semple, S. J., & Skaff, M. M. (1990). Caregiving and the stress process: An overview of concepts and their measures. *Gerontologist, 30,* 583–594.

Pearlin, L. I., & Turner, H. A. (1995). The family as a context of the stress process. In S. V. Kasl & C. L. Cooper (Eds.), *Stress and health: Issues in research methodology* (pp. 143–165). New York: Wiley.

Raudenbush, S. W., Brennan, R. T., & Barnett, R. C. (1995). A multivariate hierarchical model for studying psychological change within married couples. *Journal of Family Psychology, 9,* 161–174.

Repetti, R. L. (1989). Effects of daily workload on subsequent behavior during marital interaction: The roles of social withdrawal and spouse support. *Journal of Personality and Social Psychology, 57,* 651–659.

Sarason, I. G., Johnson, J. H., & Siegel, J. M. (1978). Assessing the impact of life changes: Development of the Life Experiences Survey. *Journal of Consulting and Clinical Psychology, 46,* 932–946.

South, S. J. (2001). The geographic context of divorce: Do neighborhoods matter? *Journal of Marriage and the Family, 63,* 755–766.

Tesser, A., & Beach, S. R. H. (1998). Life events, relationship quality, and depression: An investigation of judgment discontinuity in vivo. *Journal of Personality and Social Psychology, 74,* 36–52.

Thompson, A., & Bolger, N. (1999). Emotional transmission in couples under stress. *Journal of Marriage and the Family, 61,* 38–48.

Turner, R. J., & Wheaton, B. (1997). Checklist measurement of stressful life events. In S. Cohen, R. C. Kessler, & L. U. Gordon (Eds.), *Measuring stress: A guide for health and social scientists* (pp. 29–58). New York: Oxford University Press.

2

Dyadic Coping and Its Significance for Marital Functioning

Guy Bodenmann

For a long time, the constructs of stress and coping have been defined on an individual level. Among different stress theories, Lazarus' transactional approach (Lazarus, 1999; Lazarus & Folkman; 1984) became one of the most important, influencing a large body of research and theoretical conceptualization. Within this paradigm, stress is viewed as an interaction between demands on a person and his or her individual and social resources. Although it is an individually centered approach, this paradigm incorporates aspects of the person's social environment, although they are not explicitly stated by Lazarus. An even greater focus on aspects of the social environment is provided in Hobfoll's Conservation of Resources (CoR) approach (e.g., Hobfoll, Dunahoo, Ben-Porath, & Monnier, 1994). According to CoR theory, subjective perceptions of stress are embedded in a social context and individual coping often has social consequences.

A genuine definition of couples' coping emerged only in the early 1990s, when researchers began thinking seriously about extending the stress and coping paradigm to committed couples, families, and communities. Terms such as *dyadic stress* and *dyadic coping* appeared with reference to marital couples (see Bodenmann, 2000, for an overview). Dyadic stress and coping are defined as parts of an interpersonal process involving both marital partners. Dyadic stress is defined as a specific stressful encounter that affects both partners either directly or indirectly and triggers the coping efforts of both partners within a defined time frame and a defined geographic location. If married individuals are embedded within a shared social context, dyadic coping assumes that three elements—the interdependence of the spouses, their common concerns, and their mutual goals—stimulate a joint problem-solving process and common, emotion-focused coping activities. Dyadic coping occurs in addition to individual coping efforts (Bodenmann, 1995, 1997).

In this chapter, I begin with an examination of the concept of dyadic stress and how it impacts a couple's relationship. I then present a conceptualization of dyadic coping that builds on Lazarus' transactional stress theory by emphasizing dyadic, interpersonal, and process-oriented aspects of coping. I continue by describing forms of dyadic coping and presenting empirical evidence supporting the relation between dyadic coping and marital functioning.

This research was supported by two research grants from the Swiss National Science Foundation.

Dyadic Stress

Dyadic stress represents a distinct form of social stress. It involves common concerns, emotional intimacy between two people, and the continuity of a social system (i.e., the maintenance of the marriage). Bodenmann (1995) defined dyadic stress as a stressful event or encounter that always concerns both partners, either directly or indirectly. Thus, dyadic stress can be classified along three dimensions: (a) the way each partner is affected by the stressful event (i.e., directly or indirectly); (b) the origin of stress (i.e., whether it originates from inside or outside of the couple); and (c) the time sequence (at what moment in the coping process each partner becomes involved).

Direct and Indirect Dyadic Stress

The first dimension of dyadic stress involves whether the stressor is experienced directly or indirectly. As most marital partners spend a great deal of their day apart, each person may encounter stressors that are not directly related to the partner's daily life or to the marital relationship. In some cases, such external stressors might not affect the dyadic system when the partner to whom it occurred has handled it adequately before meeting the other partner. However, if the stressor is not coped with effectively, the stressed partner brings his or her stress home, which is likely to have a negative impact on the other partner and the marriage; for example, stress in the workplace spills over into the marital dyad (Bolger, DeLongis, Kessler, & Wethington, 1989; Repetti, 1989; Schulz, Cowan, Cowan, & Brennan, 2004). Indirect stress means that first one partner experiences stress alone (outside of the marriage) and only later the other partner, though not directly involved in the stressful event, is concerned, either by being affected by the distress of the partner (i.e., stress contagion) or when the stressed partner expresses his or her stress (verbally or nonverbally) and triggers supportive dyadic coping.

At other times, both partners face a common stressor, called *direct dyadic stress*. Although individual appraisals of this stressor occur, both partners may subsequently share a common view of it, perhaps because of the couple's shared history (see Reiss, 1981). Direct dyadic stress is defined as a stressor that affects both partners more or less at the same time (e.g., the birth of a child or moving to a new home) though sometimes in a different manner. For example, the lung cancer diagnosis of one partner concerns both partners simultaneously, but they may experience it and cope very differently. The cancer patient faces pain, treatments, limitations, and a high probability of death, whereas the partner faces caregiving stress and the potential loss of the partner.

Origin of the Stress

A second dimension of dyadic stress involves the origin of the stress, whether the stressor results from within the couple's relationship or from some event external to the couple. Stressors that originate from within the couple include differing goals, attitudes, and desires; shared problems (e.g., health problems or worries about the partner); or marital conflict. Stressors that originate outside the couple involve problems that each partner encounters individually in his or her social environment, such as those involving neighbors, extended families, or the workplace.

Time Sequence

The third dimension of dyadic stress concerns the timing of the stressors. Stress can affect both partners simultaneously or sequentially. For example, a rent increase may affect both partners simultaneously. Stress experienced in the workplace by one partner that spills over into home life is an example of sequential stress. Another example of sequential stress occurs when the coping response of one partner becomes a stressor for the other (e.g., one partner's excessive alcohol consumption). Knowledge about time sequences may be important for understanding how and when individual and dyadic coping come into play.

A Theory of Dyadic Coping

Dyadic coping has been conceptualized in a number of ways in previous research.

1. *As individual coping efforts in the context of a marriage.* This approach conceptualizes stress, even marital stress, on an individual level, something that is mastered independently by each partner alone (e.g., Pearlin & Schooler, 1978; Wolf, 1987).

2. *As an interaction between each partner's individual coping efforts.* This approach analyzes each partner's coping efforts with regard to the coping efforts of the other person (e.g., Barbarin, 1983; Barbarin, Hughes, & Chesler, 1985; Pakenham, 1998). The coping of one partner is not independent of the other partner's coping and neither is the outcome (Berghuis & Stanton, 2002). Revenson (1994, 2003, chap. 7, this volume) conceptualizes dyadic coping attempts along the dimension of congruence or incongruence; more congruent coping efforts occur when both partners cope in a similar or complementary fashion and more incongruent coping is characterized by coping strategies that are different and impede joint coping efforts.

3. *As the coping efforts of each partner focused on better functioning of the other partner and the relationship.* Approaches such as relationship-focused coping (Coyne & Smith, 1991, 1994) or empathic coping (DeLongis & O'Brien, 1990; O'Brien & DeLongis, 1997; chap. 3, this volume) focus on the well-being of the marital relationship as well as the well-being of the individual partners. They examine the coping efforts of one partner that are intended to reinforce or strengthen the psychological, physical, and social functioning of the other partner or to increase marital satisfaction. Coyne and his colleagues (Coyne & Smith, 1991, 1994; Coyne, Rohrbaugh, Shoham, Sonnega, Nicklas, &

Cranford, 2001) describe two types of relationship-focused coping, "active engagement" (involving the partner in a discussion, exploring his or her emotions, and initiating constructive attempts of problem solving), and "protective buffering" (relieving the partner emotionally, negating and minimizing worries, suppressing anger, and giving in). These concepts have been used by other researchers as well (Kuijer, Ybema, Buunk, Thijs-Boer, & Sanderman, 2000; Suls, Green, Rose, Lounsbury, & Gordon, 1997).

4. *As a dyadic coping process in which both partners are involved.* My approach (Bodenmann, 1990, 1995, 1997, 2000) is based on the trans-actional stress theory of Lazarus and Folkman (1984) but expands this theory to systemic and process-oriented dimensions. The concept of dyadic coping was first developed with regard to coping with daily hassles (minor stressors) and later expanded to critical life events (major stressors) and chronic stress in everyday life (minor stress of long duration, e.g., chronic stress at work).

In my theory of dyadic coping, a stress communication process, depicted in Figure 2.1, triggers both partners' coping responses. One partner's appraisal of a stress is communicated to the other partner, who perceives, interprets, and decodes these signals and responds with some form of dyadic coping (which might involve either acting on or ignoring the stress communication). Stress appraisals can be communicated verbally or nonverbally. Problem-focused stress is often expressed verbally, whereas emotion-focused stress may be communicated verbally or nonverbally, including voice tone, sighs, or facial expressions.

Several cognitive appraisals comprise the stress communication process: who has initially perceived the stressor (Partner A, Partner B, or both partners); what caused the stressor (the partner, others, or external causes); responsibility (e.g., guilt of the partner); and controllability (by Partner A, Partner B, or both). Depending on the stressor under consideration and what is at stake for the individual and for the marital dyad, both partners will make efforts to maintain or restore a state of homeostasis as individuals, as a couple, and with regard to other people in the couple's social world. Good adjustment is defined as either a return to prestressor functioning or personal and dyadic growth.

Several assumptions underlie this theory of dyadic coping. First, dyadic stress and coping must be conceptualized from a systems perspective. One cannot examine one partner's stress appraisals or coping efforts without con-sidering the effects on the other partner and the marriage (system). One partner's well-being and satisfaction depends on the other's well-being and satisfaction (mutual influence). Thus, both partners should be motivated to help one another deal with stressful encounters and to engage in a joint effort to deal with any stressors concerning both partners. Second, dyadic coping is only one way that the stressor is managed; individual coping efforts and sup-portive transactions (between one partner and his or her social network or between the couple and their social network) are also modes of stress man-agement. Third, dyadic coping is used most often after individual coping

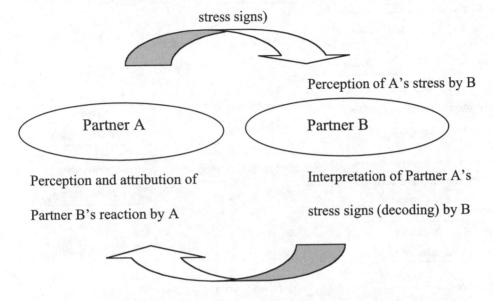

Communication of stress by Partner A

(sending verbal, nonverbal, and/or para-verbal

stress signs)

Partner A   Partner B

Perception of A's stress by B

Perception and attribution of   Interpretation of Partner A's

Partner B's reaction by A   stress signs (decoding) by B

Reaction of Partner B. There are different possibilities: (1)

no appraisal of A's stress by B (ignorance of stress by lack

of competencies or motivation), (2) stress contagion

(Partner B reacts also with stress and thus both partners are

stressed in consequence), or (3) positive or negative dyadic

coping of Partner B.

Figure 2.1. Interaction between stress communication of one partner and dyadic coping of the other one.

efforts have been made and failed. Fourth, dyadic coping involves both positive and negative modes of coping.

Forms of Dyadic Coping

Three forms of coping with stress in close relationships can be distinguished: (a) individual coping, (b) dyadic coping, and (c) seeking social support from others (e.g., friends and relatives). Dyadic coping has both positive and negative forms (see Figure 2.2). Positive forms of dyadic coping include

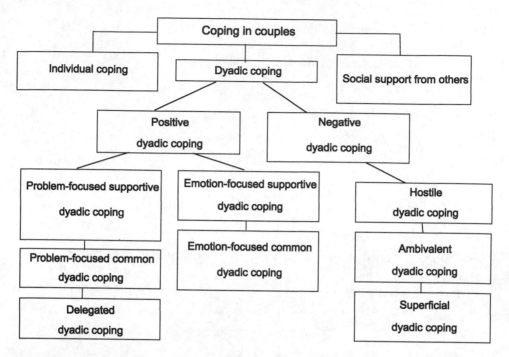

Figure 2.2.   Forms of coping in couples and differentiation of dyadic coping.

positive supportive dyadic coping, common dyadic coping, and *delegated dyadic coping.* Positive supportive and common dyadic coping may be either problem focused or emotion focused. Negative forms of dyadic coping include *hostile, ambivalent,* and *superficial* dyadic coping. Each of the forms of positive and negative dyadic coping is described in the paragraphs that follow.

Positive supportive dyadic coping occurs when one partner assists the other in his or her coping efforts. This can be expressed through activities such as helping with daily tasks or providing practical advice, empathic understanding, helping the partner to reframe the situation, communicating a belief in the partner's capabilities, or expressing solidarity with the partner ("This reaction would also hurt me if I were in this situation"). Positive supportive dyadic coping is not simply altruistic behavior but involves efforts to support the partner that have the secondary goal of reducing one's own stress as well (Bodenmann, 1995). Because the unresolved or ineffectively handled stress of one partner affects the other, both partners have a vital interest in supporting one another in order to guarantee their own well-being as well as the well-being and stability of their relationship.

In common dyadic coping, both partners participate in the coping process more or less symmetrically or complementarily in order to handle a problem-focused or emotion-focused issue relevant to the dyad by using strategies such as joint problem solving, joint information seeking, sharing of feelings, mutual commitment, or relaxing together. Whereas supportive dyadic coping means that one partner helps the other to deal with stress, in common dyadic coping both partners are experiencing stress (often because of the same stressor, i.e., direct dyadic stress) and try to manage the situation by coping jointly. They apply strategies focusing on resolving the problem together or helping each other reduce emotional arousal.

Delegated dyadic coping occurs when one partner takes over responsibilities in order to reduce the stress experienced by his or her mate. As opposed to supportive dyadic coping, during delegated dyadic coping, the partner is explicitly asked to give support and a new division of contributions to the coping process is established. This form of dyadic coping is most commonly used in response to problem-oriented stressors. For example, the partner who doesn't usually do food shopping does the shopping in order to reduce the partner's stress.

Negative forms of dyadic coping include *hostile dyadic coping*, which involves support that is accompanied by disparagement, distancing, mocking or sarcasm, open disinterest, or minimizing the seriousness of the partner's stress. This means that the supporting partner provides help (e.g., gives advice) but does so in a negative way. These reactions are not to be confounded with negative communication behavior (see Gottman, 1994), as support is provided but it is accompanied by hostile elements, often on the paraverbal or nonverbal level. *Ambivalent dyadic coping* occurs when one partner supports the other unwillingly or with the attitude that his or her contribution should be unnecessary. *Superficial dyadic coping* consists of support that is insincere, for example, asking questions about the partner's feelings without listening or supporting the partner without empathy.

Dyadic coping is shaped and maintained by individual and dyadic appraisals, common goals, and shared resources (Bodenmann, 1995). Positive supportive dyadic coping and delegated dyadic coping are triggered by the appraisal of the supporting partner that the stress was not directly caused by the partner and the appraisal of one's own resources as sufficient to support the partner. For example, if the husband sees that his wife has not caused the stressful event and thinks he is able to help, he is more likely to engage in positive supportive or delegated dyadic coping. All types of dyadic coping are influenced by a number of intra- and extrapersonal factors: *individual skills*, such as stress communication skills, problem-solving skills, social competence, and organizational skills; *motivational factors*, such as relationship satisfaction or interest in the longevity of the relationship; and *contextual factors*, such as the current level of stress experienced by both partners or their current moods.

It is important to distinguish the construct of dyadic coping from that of social support (Bodenmann, 1995). First, social support received from the partner has a different meaning than support received from friends and relatives. Many studies reveal that the support from the partner is of primary significance and represents the most important source of support (e.g., Revenson, 1994), and motivational factors vary with regard to social support provided to friends or to partners (Veiel, Crisand, Stroszeck-Somschor, & Herrle, 1991; Williamson & Clark, 1992). Second, dyadic coping is not an altruistic behavior but an engagement of both partners in order to assure the partners' satisfaction and well-being, which in turn assures one's own marital satisfaction and well-being. When a partner is able to reduce stress for the other partner, negative influences on the relationship are reduced and positive outcomes are more likely (see also, the negative-state-relief hypothesis; Cialdini, Darby, & Vincent, 1973). Third, social support is only one form of dyadic coping, additional ones are common dyadic coping and delegated dyadic coping.

The Stress-Coping Cascade

A stress-coping cascade (see Figure 2.3) is triggered when one or both partners makes a stress appraisal (Bodenmann, 2000); that is, the process of coping follows a dynamic temporal order. In the majority of cases, both partners usually try individual strategies in their first attempts at coping with a stressful encounter. When individual coping efforts are not successful in managing the stressor, dyadic coping is brought into play. If dyadic coping efforts are not successful, social support from outside of the couple may be required to handle the stressful situation. When individual, dyadic, and social coping efforts do not bring relief, professional help may be sought (see also the different stages of stress described by Burr & Klein, 1994). However, this temporal progression is not fixed in stone; if one partner experiences a particular stress related to work, then he or she might activate social support from coworkers before consulting a spouse.

Partial evidence for the stress-coping cascade is provided in a study of 98 Swiss community-residing couples (Bodenmann, 2000). Most often only indi-

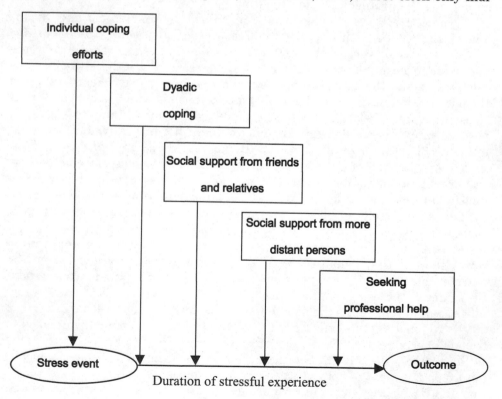

Figure 2.3. Stress-coping cascade in close relationships: the process of coping in couples.

vidual coping was displayed at the beginning of a stressful episode, followed by dyadic coping, and later by social support. Social support was often sought by women at an earlier stage than by men. New coping resources did not replace existing ones but added to them. Thus, individuals continued to cope individually or on the dyadic level (although in a reduced way) when social support from friends or relatives was received. Moreover, the more severe the stressor was or the longer it persisted, the more coping resources that were activated (in the postulated order).

The Significance of Dyadic Coping for Relationship Functioning

Dyadic coping has two primary objectives: the reduction of stress for each partner and the enhancement of relationship quality. One partner's well-being depends on the other's well-being, as well as his or her integration within the social environment. In situations in which one partner's individual coping resources are insufficient or both partners are confronted with the same stressful event, dyadic coping should help to manage stress for both partners. However, positive dyadic coping has a second and equally important effect on the relationship: It fosters a feeling of *we-ness*—that is, mutual trust, reliability, commitment, and the perception that the relationship is a supportive resource in difficult circumstances (see also chaps. 4, 6, & 9, this volume; Cutrona, 1996). In addition to its stress reduction goals, dyadic coping is an important factor in maintaining or enhancing marital quality and stability (Bodenmann, 2000).

Empirical Findings on Dyadic Coping and Its Significance for Marital Functioning

Bodenmann and his colleagues have collected data from over 1,200 couples with regard to dyadic coping and its role in marital functioning. We have conducted both intervention and observational–correlational studies, using cross-sectional and longitudinal designs and multiple methods of data collection, including self-report questionnaires, written diaries, a stress-coping interview, and systematic observation in both laboratory and field settings. In addition, we carried out three intervention studies in order to evaluate the effectiveness of a dyadic-coping intervention, the Couples Coping Enhancement Training (Bodenmann & Shantinath, 2004), described in chapter 8 of this volume.

We conducted a meta-analysis on the relationship between dyadic coping and marital satisfaction across 13 studies that included a total of 783 couples who were either legally married or in a long-term intimate relationship. Eleven studies were of community-residing adults who had answered an advertisement to participate in marital research, and two studies involved clinical samples recruited in clinics and private practices, one study in which one partner had an anxiety disorder (Schütz, 1999) and one study in which one partner had a depressive disorder (Schwerzmann, 2000). One of the studies of community-residing adults was of lesbian couples (Kunz, 1997); the other 12 studies involved heterosexual relationships. None of the studies in the meta-analysis included any couples who had participated in a marital intervention. All but one of the studies used the Fragebogen zur Erfassung des Dyadischen Copings als Tendenz (FDCT-N; Bodenmann, 1990)[1] as the measure of dyadic coping; the exception (Wüst, 1997) used a stress-coping interview format that was subsequently coded for the six forms of dyadic coping described earlier. Marital satisfaction was assessed by the Partnerschaftsfragebogen (PFB; Hahlweg, 1996) in eight of the studies and the Marital Needs Satisfaction Scale (Stinnet, Collins, & Montgomery, 1970) in five of the studies.

The results of the meta-analysis are presented in Table 2.1. The overall effect size, $d = 1.3$, provides convincing evidence of a relationship between dyadic coping and marital functioning. In all 13 studies, positive dyadic coping was associated significantly with better marital functioning and higher relationship satisfaction, with dyadic coping accounting for 30% to 40% of the variance in marital satisfaction. In all 13 studies, we found higher scores on the measure of positive dyadic coping among couples higher in marital satisfaction compared with distressed couples, who displayed more negative dyadic coping (ambivalent, hostile, or superficial dyadic coping). In addition, significantly higher scores on negative dyadic coping were found for the clinical couples compared with couples in community samples (Bodenmann, 2000).

The association between dyadic coping and relationship functioning also was supported by observational data using microanalytic coding (Bodenmann, 1990, 1995, 2000). In a study of 63 married Swiss community-residing couples, positive dyadic coping behavior was significantly higher among couples with high marital satisfaction. Couples higher in marital satisfaction demonstrated greater problem- and emotion-focused stress communication and supportive dyadic coping (such as empathy and attention, verbal emotion-focused supportive dyadic coping, and emotion-focused common dyadic coping) and less negative dyadic coping (hostile and superficial dyadic coping) than less satisfied couples (Bodenmann, 2000).

Other evidence supporting the relation between dyadic coping and martial satisfaction was found in an experimental study conducted in a laboratory (Bodenmann, 1995, 2000). Seventy couples were videotaped for 10 minutes in two identical settings, once before and once after an experimental stress induction. Both observational and self-report data showed that couples experiencing stress communicated an increased number of verbal and nonverbal stress signals to the partner and that all forms of dyadic coping increased under stress.

Our data also provide evidence of a long-term association between dyadic coping and marital functioning. A 5-year longitudinal study examined the effects of dyadic stress on relationship quality and stability (Bodenmann & Cina, 2000). Dyadic coping was among the most powerful predictors for sepa-

---

[1]We developed and validated a self-report questionnaire, *Fragebogen zur Erfassung des Dyadischen Copings als Tendenz* (FDCT-N) to measure these forms of dyadic coping. The FDCT-N consists of 41 items that are answered individually by each partner. There is also a diary version of the questionnaire and a stress-coping interview and microanalytic behavioral coping system (Bodenmann, 2000). Information about the FDCT-N and its psychometric properties can be found in Bodenmann (1990, 2000).

Table 2.1. Meta-Analysis of 13 Studies Examining the Relation Between Dyadic Coping and Marital Satisfaction

Study	Sample characteristics				Measure		Correlation between coping and marital satisfaction ($p < .001$)
	N (couples)	Age (SD)	Nationality	Community-residing (CO) or clinical (CL)	Dyadic coping	Marital satisfaction	
Alderisi (1996)	20	37.5 (9.8)	Italian	CO	FDCT	PFB	.53
Backman (1996)	40	34.8 (9.4)	French	CO	FDCT	MNS	.51
Bodenmann (1990)	22	27.8 (8.2)	Swiss	CO	FDCT	MNS	.54
Bodenmann (1995)	70	29.7 (7.3)	Swiss	CO	FDCT	MNS	.52
Bodenmann (1995)	220	40.1 (9.1)	Swiss	CO	FDCT	PFB	.67
Bodenmann (2000)	22	30.7 (6.6)	Swiss	CO	FDCT	MNS	.59
Freudiger (1995)	79	35.5 (7.6)	Swiss	CO	FDCT	PFB	.58
Kunz (1997)	38	50.9 (15.8)	Swiss	CO	FDCT	MNS	.63
Maurer (1995)	48	36.9 (15.1)	Swiss	CO	FDCT	PFB	.52
Senti (1996)	74	41.5 (9.9)	Swiss	CL	FDCT	PFB	.57
Schütz (1999)				(anxiety disorder)			
	60	43.2 (9.3)	Swiss	CL	FDCT	PFB	.52
Schwerzmann (2000)				(depressive disorder)			
Tafra (1996)	56	30.9 (8.9)	Swiss	CO	FDCT	PFB	.36
Wüst (1997)	34	33.7 (10.0)	Swiss	CO	interview	PFB	.66

Note. FDCT-N = total score of the *Fragebogen zur Erfassung des Dyadischen Copings als Tendenz* (Bodenmann, 1990); PFB = total score of the *Partnerschaftsfragebogen* (Partnership Questionnaire, Hahlweg, 1996); MNS = total score of the *Marital Needs Satisfaction Scale* (Stinnet et al., 1970).

ration and divorce at 1-, 2-, 3-, and 5-year follow-ups. Looking retrospectively, we found that couples high in marital satisfaction at the end of the study displayed more positive supportive dyadic coping (i.e., problem- and emotion-focused supportive coping) and common dyadic coping at earlier times than did couples who were separated or divorced by the 5-year follow-up. Entering only the Time 1 stress and coping variables into a discriminant function analysis, we were able to predict three groups of couples with 62% accuracy: stable and satisfied; stable and unsatisfied; and separated or divorced. Stable satisfied couples were couples who, at the 5-year follow-up, were still together and rated their marital quality as high. Stable unsatisfied couples stayed together but rated their marital quality as low. When only two discriminant functions were assessed, stable versus divorced couples, 73% of the couples were correctly classified.

How Does Dyadic Coping Affect the Relationship Between Stress and Marital Quality?

Numerous authors have shown that stress is inversely correlated with marital satisfaction (Blood & Wolfe, 1965; Bodenmann, 2000; Burke & Weir, 1977; Wolf, 1987; Neff & Karney, 2004). It is noteworthy that the nature of the stressor (life events vs. daily hassles vs. developmental transitions) has different effects on the marital relationship. Chronic stressors (i.e., persistent daily hassles) have been associated with lower marital satisfaction (see chap. 1, this volume). Life event stressors, in contrast, have not been correlated with marital satisfaction unless the life events involve ongoing close relationships, including severe marital distress, heavy conflicts with the partner, separation, or divorce (Williams, 1995). And in some marriages, life events may enhance marital cohesion (McCubbin & Patterson, 1983). It is possible that in these cases, partners provide mutual support and engage in dyadic coping, appraising the stressful event as a dyadic stressor that challenges *both* partners. Thus, the partners' appraisals of who is affected by the stressful event and whether the stressor is defined as an individual or relationship problem may be determinants of marital outcomes.

How does stress affect marriage? In an earlier book (Bodenmann, 2000), I argued that chronic everyday stress affects close relationships in multiple ways, as illustrated in Figure 2.4. First, stress can minimize the time partners spend together, reducing opportunities for common experiences, mutual emotional self-disclosure, tenderness, and satisfying sexuality and lowering the feeling of *we-ness* of the couple. For example, partners who experience high job stress often spend more time in the office, work longer hours, or bring work home. As a consequence, they are less emotionally available, including less emotional self-disclosure, less time for common experiences and shared moments, and less time for dyadic coping. An exception to this is major life events. For example, couples coping with a serious illness, such as cancer, may actually spend more time together if the patient is at home more (see chap. 9, this volume). In these cases, the stressor provides an opportunity to become closer.

A second way that stress affects marriage is to decrease the quality of dyadic communication. As Bodenmann (1995) has shown in an experimental

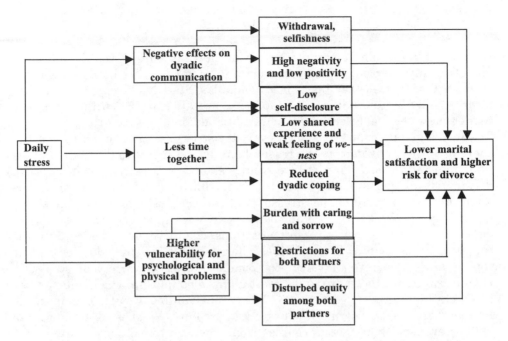

Figure 2.4. Relationship between chronic daily stress and marital functioning.

laboratory study, the quality of marital communication declined under conditions of stress by as much as 40% (see also Conger, Ge, & Lorenz, 1994; Crouter, Perry-Jerkins, Huston, & Crawford, 1989; Kinnunen & Pulkkinen, 1998; Repetti, 1989). When partners were stressed they displayed more negative communication patterns (criticism, domineering, contempt, belligerence, and withdrawal), which are predictors of poor marital functioning and a higher risk of divorce (Gottman, 1994; Weiss & Heyman, 1997).

Third, chronic stress may increase the risk of physical and psychological health problems (Goldberger & Breznitz, 1982). Chronic stress reduces opportunities for pleasant activities and challenges equity of roles between the partners. As a consequence, marital satisfaction is reduced (Burman & Margolin, 1992; Manne & Zautra, 1990). Occasionally, chronic stressors originating outside of the marriage go unnoticed or are underestimated by one or both of the partners. This may gradually erode the relationship without the couple realizing it. This spill-over of stress originating outside of the relationship leads to a more superficial kind of dyadic interaction, involving less of the partner's emotional needs. Feelings of alienation (either individual or mutual) may become the source of more frequent marital conflicts, and in the long run, increase marital distress. However, the more effectively each partner copes with his or her own stress, the more he or she can reduce the likelihood of spill-over, and thereby, protect the relationship from the negative effects of stress. The same is true for dyadic coping. Engaging in positive dyadic coping by jointly discussing the stress experience, reframing the situation, or helping each other to relax increases a sense of solidarity or *we-ness* and is likely to reduce stress, and in so doing, promote marital happiness and cohesion. Individual and dyadic coping are thus seen as protective factors for marital functioning.

Conclusion

Dyadic coping is an important new concept that goes beyond traditional models of interpersonal communication and social support in close relationships. Stress in everyday life is not avoidable; thus, dyadic coping is of vital interest. The better that partners *together* are able to cope with stress, the higher their chance for optimal marital satisfaction and stability.

Although our knowledge about everyday stress and dyadic coping is solid, there are still many gaps in the research on dyadic coping and research questions to be addressed. First, future studies should make stronger attempts to distinguish among different types of stress that couples face and to understand how the nature of the stressor and the couples' appraisal of it shape dyadic coping. We know little about how partners' appraisal processes influence each other and how stressful situations, cognitive variables, and dyadic coping are associated. Second, researchers should explore whether dyadic coping processes have universal components across a variety of stressors. Dyadic coping has been examined most often in couples in which one partner has a chronic illness (e.g., chaps. 6, 7, & 9, this volume; Coyne, Thompson, & Palmer, 2002; Hagedoorn, Kuijer, Buunk, DeJong, Wobbes, & Sanderman, 2000; Revenson, 2003), or in couples from community samples dealing with everyday stress (e.g., Bodenmann, 2000). Little research has explored dyadic coping among couples in which one partner suffers from a mental health problem (for an exception, see Bodenmann, Widmer, Charvoz, & Bradbury, 2004). Third, it is our hope that as research continues in this area, constructs will be defined more clearly and measurement tools will become more precise.

We are convinced that dyadic coping is not only an intriguing theoretical concept but it is also of clinical importance. To improve the way couples cope together is an important target of cognitive behavioral therapy as is prevention of marital dissatisfaction. We believe that interventions focusing on improving dyadic coping (e.g., Couples Coping Enhancement Training, CCET; Bodenmann & Shantinath, 2004) add value to current modalities in marital distress prevention training or marital therapy. The question of how couples cope together in addition to their individual coping efforts and social support from their network merits much greater interest than it has received thus far.

References

Alderisi, S. (1996). *Alltagsbelastungen, dyadisches Coping und social Support* [Daily stress, dyadic coping and social support]. Unpublished master's thesis, University of Fribourg, Fribourg, Switzerland.

Backman, H. (1996). *Satisfaction, communication et gestion du stress de différents types de couples* [Satisfaction, communication and dyadic coping in different kind of couples]. Unpublished master's thesis, University of Fribourg, Fribourg, Switzerland.

Barbarin, O. A. (1983). Coping with ecological transitions by Black families: A psychosocial model. *Journal of Community Psychology, 11,* 308–322.

Barbarin, O. A., Hughes, D., & Chesler, M. A. (1985). Stress, coping, and marital functioning among partners of children with cancer. *Journal of Marriage and the Family, 47,* 473–480.

Berghuis, J. P., & Stanton, A. L. (2002). Adjustment to a dyadic stressor: A longitudinal study of coping and depressive symptoms in infertile couples over an insemination attempt. *Journal of Consulting and Clinical Psychology, 70,* 433–438.

Blood, R. O., & Wolfe, D. M. (1965). *Husbands and wives: The dynamics of married living.* Glencoe, IL: Free Press.

Bodenmann, G. (1990). *Ärgerregulation und deren Bedeutung für die dyadische Interaktion* [Anger regulation and its significance for dyadic interaction]. Fribourg, Switzerland: University of Fribourg.

Bodenmann, G. (1995). A systemic-transactional conceptualization of stress and coping in couples. *Swiss Journal of Psychology, 54,* 34–49.

Bodenmann, G. (1997). Dyadic coping—a systemic-transactional view of stress and coping among couples: Theory and empirical findings. *European Review of Applied Psychology, 47,* 137–140.

Bodenmann, G. (2000). *Stress und Coping bei Paaren* [Stress and coping in couples]. Göttingen, Germany: Hogrefe.

Bodenmann, G., & Cina, A. (2000). Stress und Coping als Prädiktoren für Scheidung: Eine prospektive Fünf-Jahres-Längsschnittstudie [Stress and coping as predictors of divorce: A 5-year prospective longitudinal study]. *Zeitschrift für Familienforschung, 12,* 5–20.

Bodenmann, G., & Shantinath, S. D. (2004). The Couples Coping Enhancement Training (CCET): A new approach to prevention of marital distress based upon stress and coping. *Family Relations, 53,* 477–484.

Bodenmann, G., Widmer, K., Charvoz, L., & Bradbury, T. N. (2004). Differences in individual and dyadic coping in depressed, non-depressed and remitted persons. *Journal of Psychopathology and Behavioral Assessment, 26,* 75–85.

Bolger, N., DeLongis, A., Kessler, R. C., & Wethington, E. (1989). The contagion of stress across multiple roles. *Journal of Marriage and the Family, 51,* 175–183.

Burke, R. J., & Weir, T. (1977). Marital helping relationships: The moderators between stress and well-being. *The Journal of Psychology, 95,* 121–130.

Burman, B., & Margolin, G. (1992). Analysis of the association between marital relationships and health problems: An interactional perspective. *Psychological Bulletin, 112,* 39–63.

Burr, W. R., & Klein, S. (Eds.). (1994). *Managing family stress.* Newbury Park, CA: Sage.

Cialdini, R. B., Darby, B. L., & Vincent, J. E. (1973). Transgression and altruism: A case for hedonism. *Journal of Experimental Social Psychology, 9,* 502–516.

Conger, R. D., Ge, X. J., & Lorenz, F. O. (1994). Economic stress and marital relationships. In R. D. Conger & G. H. Elder (Eds.), *Families in troubled times* (pp. 187–203). New York: Walter de Gruyter.

Coyne, J. C., Rohrbaugh, M. J., Shoham, V., Sonnega, J., Nicklas, J. M., & Cranford, J. A. (2001). Prognostic importance of marital quality for survival of congestive heart failure. *American Journal of Cardiology, 88,* 526–529.

Coyne, J. C., & Smith, D. A. F. (1991). Couples coping with a myocardial infarction: A contextual perspective on wives' distress. *Journal of Personality and Social Psychology, 61,* 404–412.

Coyne, J. C., & Smith, D. A. F. (1994). Couples coping with myocardial infarction: Contextual perspective on patient self-efficacy. *Journal of Family Psychology, 8,* 1–13.

Coyne, J. C., Thompson, R., & Palmer, S. (2002). Marital quality, coping with conflicts, marital complaints, and affection in couples with a depressed wife. *Journal of Family Psychology, 16,* 26–37.

Crouter, A. C., Perry-Jerkins, M., Huston, T. L., & Crawford, D. W. (1989). The influence of work-induced psychological states on behavior at home. *Basic and Applied Social Psychology, 10,* 273–292.

Cutrona, C. E. (1996). *Social support in couples. Marriage as a resource in times of stress.* Thousand Oaks, CA: Sage.

DeLongis, A., & O'Brien, T. B. (1990). An interpersonal framework for stress and coping: An application to the families of Alzheimer's patients. In M. A. P. Stephens, J. H. Crowther, S. E. Hobfoll, & D. L. Tennenbaum (Eds.), *Stress and coping in later-life families* (pp. 221–239). New York: Hemisphere Publication Services.

Freudiger, M. (1995). *Problembewältigung und Dominanz in Partnerschaften* [Problem-solving and dominance in close relationships]. Unpublished master's thesis, University of Fribourg, Fribourg, Switzerland.

Goldberger, L., & Breznitz, S. (Eds.). (1982). *Handbook of stress: Theoretical and clinical aspects.* New York: The Free Press.

Gottman, J. M. (1994). *What predicts divorce?* Hillsdale, NJ: Erlbaum.

Hagedoorn, M., Kuijer, R. G., Buunk, B. P., DeJong, G. M., Wobbes, T., & Sanderman, R. (2000). Marital satisfaction in patients with cancer: Does support from intimate partners benefit those who need it the most? *Health Psychology, 19,* 274–282.

Hahlweg, K. (1996). *Fragebogen zur Partnerschaftsdiagnostik (FPD)* [Partnership Questionnaire]. Göttingen, Germany: Hogrefe.

Hobfoll, S. E., Dunahoo, C. A., Ben-Porath, Y., & Monnier, J. (1994). Gender and coping: The dual axis model of coping. *American Journal of Community Psychology, 22,* 49–82.

Kinnunen, U., & Pulkkinen, L. (1998). Linking economic stress to marital quality among Finnish marital couples. *Journal of Family Issues, 19,* 705–724.

Kuijer, R. G., Ybema, J. F., Buunk, B. P., Thijs-Boer, F., & Sanderman, R. (2000). Active engagement, protective buffering, and overprotection: Three ways of giving support by intimate partners of patients with cancer. *Journal of Social and Clinical Psychology, 19,* 256–285.

Kunz, B. (1997). *Partnerinnenzufriedenheit, Belastung und Belastungsbewältigung bei lesbischen Paaren* [Relationship satisfaction, stress and coping in lesbian couples]. Unpublished master's thesis, University of Fribourg, Fribourg, Switzerland.

Lazarus, R. S. (1999). *Stress and emotion.* New York: Springer Publishing Company.

Lazarus, R. S., & Folkman, S. (1984). *Stress, appraisal, and coping.* New York: Springer Publishing Company.

Manne, S. L., & Zautra, A. J. (1990). Couples coping with chronic illness: Women with rheumatoid arthritis and their healthy husbands. *Journal of Behavioral Medicine, 13,* 327–342.

Maurer, C. (1995). *Dyadische Bewältigung von Stress: Eine Altersstichprobe* [Dyadic coping in elderly couples]. Unpublished master's thesis, University of Fribourg, Fribourg, Switzerland.

McCubbin, H. I., & Patterson, J. M. (1983). The family stress process: The double ABCX-model of adjustment and adaptation. *Marriage and Family Review, 6,* 7–37.

Neff, L. A., & Karney, B. R. (2004). How does context affect intimate relationships? Linking external stress and cognitive processes within marriage. *Personality and Social Psychology Bulletin, 30,* 134–148.

O'Brien, T. B., & DeLongis, A. (1997). Coping with chronic stress: An interpersonal perspective. In B. Gottlieb (Ed.), *Coping with chronic stress* (pp. 162–190). New York: Plenum Press.

Pakenham, K. I. (1998). Couple coping and adjustment to multiple sclerosis in care receiver–carer dyads. *Family Relations, 47,* 269–277.

Pearlin, L. I., & Schooler, C. (1978). The structure of coping. *Journal of Health and Social Behavior, 19,* 2–21.

Reiss, D. (1981). *The family's construction of reality.* Cambridge, MA: Harvard University Press.

Repetti, R. L. (1989). Effects of daily workload on subsequent behavior during marital interaction: The roles of social withdrawal and spouse support. *Journal of Personality and Social Psychology, 57,* 651–659.

Revenson, T. A. (1994). Social support and marital coping with chronic illness. *Annals of Behavioural Medicine, 16,* 122–130.

Revenson, T. A. (2003). Scenes from a marriage: Examining support, coping, and gender within the context of chronic illness. In J. Suls & K. Wallston (Eds.), *Social psychological foundations of health and illness* (pp. 530–559). Oxford, England: Blackwell Publishers.

Schulz, M. S., Cowan, P. A., Cowan, C. P., & Brennan, R. T. (2004). Coming home upset: Gender, marital satisfaction, and the daily spillover of workday experience into couples interactions. *Journal of Family Psychology, 18,* 250–263.

Schütz, B. (1999). *Angst und Partnerschaft. Belastungsbewältigung von Paaren, bei denen die Frau oder der Mann an einer Angststörung leidet* [Anxiety and close relationships. Coping in couples with an anxiety disorder]. Unpublished master's thesis, University of Fribourg, Fribourg, Switzerland.

Schwerzmann, S. (2000). *Depression, stress, coping and marriage.* Unpublished master's thesis, University of Fribourg, Fribourg, Switzerland.

Senti, P. (1996). *Belastungsbewältigung in verschiedenen Partnerschaftsbereichen und ihr Zusammenhang zu Geschlechtsrollen* [Coping in different stress domains with regard to gender roles]. Unpublished master's thesis, University of Fribourg, Fribourg, Switzerland.

Stinnet, N., Collins, J., & Montgomery, J. E. (1970). Marital need satisfactions of older husbands and wives. *Journal of Marriage and the Family, 8,* 428–434.

Suls, J., Green, P., Rose, G., Lounsbury, P., & Gordon, E. (1997). Hiding worries from one's spouse: Associations between coping via protective buffering and distress in male post-myocardial infarction patients and their wives. *Journal of Behavioral Medicine, 20,* 333–349.

Tafra, R. (1996). *Die Bedeutung des hedonistischen Repertoires für die Partnerschaft und das dyadische Coping* [The significance of hedonistic activities for dyadic coping in close relationships]. Unpublished master's thesis, University of Fribourg, Fribourg, Switzerland.

Veiel, H. O. F., Crisand, M., Stroszeck-Somschor, H., & Herrle, J. (1991). Social support networks of chronically strained couples: Similarity and overlap. *Journal of Social and Personal Relationships, 8,* 279–292.

Weiss, R. L., & Heyman, R. E. (1997). A clinical overview of couples interactions. In W. K. Halford & H. J. Markman (Eds.), *Clinical handbook of marriage and couples interventions* (pp. 13–41). New York: Wiley.

Williams, L. M. (1995). Association of stressful life events and marital quality. *Psychological Reports, 76,* 1115–1122.

Williamson, G. M., & Clark, M. S. (1992). Impact of desired relationship type on affective reactions to choosing and being required to help. *Personality and Social Psychology Bulletin, 18,* 10–18.

Wolf, W. (1987). *Alltagsbelastungen und Partnerschaft.* Bern, Switzerland: Huber.

Wüst, G. (1997). *Stressverhalten in Paarbeziehungen* [Coping in close relationships: An interview approach assessing dyadic coping in couples]. Unpublished master's thesis, University of Fribourg, Fribourg, Switzerland.

3

A Contextual Examination of Stress and Coping Processes in Stepfamilies

Melady Preece and Anita DeLongis

Increasingly, researchers have become interested in stress and coping processes in close relationships. Interpersonal factors play a major role in physical and psychological well-being (Cramer, 1985; Feldman, Downey, & Schaffer-Neitz, 1999) as well as in the ability to successfully deal with stress (Kramer, 1993; O'Brien & DeLongis, 1997). Because of the unique set of interpersonal stressors with which most stepfamilies must cope, this family form provides a rich context in which to examine interpersonal stress, coping, and social support.

In this chapter, we summarize findings from our recent study of stepfamilies. First, we highlight the problems and challenges faced by stepfamilies and provide qualitative examples of key issues in these families from interviews with the participants in our study. Then, we describe findings from our study pertaining to relationship quality in stepfamilies. Next, we summarize findings from our research pertaining to the relationship between coping and relationship quality between parents and children. We have found five coping strategies to be particularly relevant to managing interpersonal stressors: empathy, support provision, compromise, confrontation, and interpersonal withdrawal. Our findings include both short-term (i.e., within the course of a single day) and long-term predictors (i.e., across 2 years) of relationship quality in stepfamilies.

Problems and Challenges of Stepfamily Life

Remarriage has the potential to positively influence the overall functioning of a family previously headed by a single parent. In the best possible scenario, the addition of a new stepparent can provide economic advantages, as well as emotional and child-rearing support, to the biological parent (Zill, Morrison, & Coiro, 1993). However, as often as not, the promise of improved family well-being goes unrealized. Members of a new stepfamily must cope with a number of stressors unique to the remarried family structure that can be so problematic as to outweigh any advantages. For example, establishing and maintaining a strong marital bond is more challenging when the stepparent must simultaneously work to construct a

This research was supported by research operating grants from the Social Science and Humanities Research Council of Canada to Anita DeLongis and a British Columbia Health Research Foundation Doctoral Fellowship to Melady Preece.

functional stepparent–stepchild relationship. Similarly, while working to develop a close marital relationship, remarried parents also need to sustain a close relationship with their children from a previous union and to resolve the loyalty conflicts that are likely to emerge (Hetherington & Jodl, 1994). As the wife in one stepfamily in our study explained:

> We have started taking separate vacations, each of us with our own kids. So there is not enough time away together. Each of us has to go alone so that the other can stay home with the other kids. I need to spend more quality time alone with my husband without the kids around.

A great deal of research suggests that stepfamilies are at increased risk for stress of all kinds (Bray & Berger, 1993; Bray & Heatherington, 1993; Hetherington, Bridges, & Insabella, 1998; Hobart, 1990; Jacobson, 1990; Wallerstein & Blakeslee, 1989). Many of these stressors are unique to stepfamilies, such as conflicting loyalties between the parent and biological children and the new spouse (Kheshgi-Genovese & Genovese, 1997; Papernow, 1987), conflicts between divorced parents (Bray & Heatherington), diminished family cohesion (Bray & Berger), the assumption of new roles and relationships that are fraught with complexity and ambiguity (McGoldrick & Carter, 1988), conflicts surrounding the distribution of financial resources between two households (Crosbie-Burnett & Ahrons, 1985; Fishman, 1983), difficulties associated with children going between two households (e.g., residential and noncustodial; Bray, 1991), and conflicts between subsystems of the stepfamily (e.g., stepparents and stepchildren, biological children and stepchildren; McGoldrick & Carter). Research indicates that stepfamilies do eventually find ways of adapting and thus diminishing their stress levels, but this may not occur until after the children have left the stepfamily home. For example, Zeppa and Norem (1993) found that the stress levels among stepfamilies become equal to the stress levels among first-family marriages by the 14th year of marriage.

Martial Satisfaction in Remarried Couples

Although marital satisfaction in first marriages tends to be higher than marital satisfaction in remarriages, the differences are quite small (Coleman & Ganong, 1990). A common theme among remarried couples in our study was that if it were not for the difficulties they have with their children and stepchildren, everything would be fine. A study investigating the effect of stepchildren on marital quality (White & Booth, 1985) found that only those remarried couples with stepchildren living in the home had divorce rates higher than those of first marriage couples. Given this, it appears that marital adjustment is most adversely affected by the presence of stepchildren and child-rearing issues (Hobart, 1991). For the most part, these issues disappear after the stepchildren leave the home.

Parent–Child Relationships in Stepfamilies

The quality of the stepparent–stepchild relationship is believed by many to be the most important relationship in predicting overall stepfamily happiness (Crosbie-Burnett, 1984; Visher & Visher, 1988). It is also the most problematic and stressful stepfamily relationship (Mills, 1984). It is well documented that stepfamilies tend to experience more interpersonal stressors than do first marriage families (Crosbie-Burnett, 1989). However, very little is known about how stepfamilies cope on a daily basis and how their ways of coping affect the quality of stepfamily relationships. Because many stepparent–stepchild relationships do not have the solid foundation created by early childhood bonding experiences, the stepparent–stepchild bond may be particularly vulnerable.

The Stepfather–Stepchild Relationship

A positive relationship between stepfathers and stepchildren can lead to positive outcomes for the child and for the family (Hetherington, 1982). Ganong and Coleman (1994) hypothesized a scenario in which a newly married mother's early preoccupation with her spouse may create feelings of jealousy and insecurity in her young children. The children may withdraw from her, create conflicts with the stepfather, or misbehave and act out in order to demand their mother's attention. Such behavior may also negatively affect the stepfather–stepchild relationship. When new stepfathers find themselves rejected in their early attempts to become involved with their stepchildren, they may withdraw from their stepchildren and relinquish the parental role. One mother described the relationship with her daughter from a previous marriage and her current husband in this way:

> I think he feels very badly that . . . he thinks she doesn't feel for him the way a natural daughter would feel for a father and in fact he has been her father for 11 years and she has very little contact with her natural father. If he had started when we were first married and she was very young, she was five, he would have been able to . . .buy her love by the way he treated her, by showing her a different kind of affection, but he wasn't willing to do that. They have a weird relationship. I know that he's very fond of her and that he's very proud of her and he loves her too but he never ever says that—never directly to her. And he'll actually very seldom praise her to her face but he's always telling other people how wonderful she is. He could tell her straight up that he cares for her and she'd feel good about that . . . but I think he'd probably choke on it before he'd say it.

As disengaged parenting of stepchildren is the predominant style of step-fathers (Hetherington, 1993), it may be that such disengagement leads to the common failure of stepchildren to adapt successfully to membership in a remarried family.

Little research has examined how mothers' behavior may impact the relationship between stepfathers and stepchildren. Indeed, the mother's behavior may affect not only stepfather–stepchild relationships but also the father's relationships with his own children. No doubt fathers' behavior also has an impact on stepmother–stepchild relationships, as we discuss below in the section on stepmothers.

One wife described some typical problems that can arise when both parents have children. She identified that the major issue in their family involved her stepson's rude and inconsiderate behavior contrasted with her husband's view that she tended to coddle her own son. Two years later she described how the problem had grown, stating that her husband wanted her to be available for his children, but he would not contribute an equal amount of effort and concern for her children. She stated that he maintained a distance from her children and resented the closeness she had with her children. It is not surprising that her husband had a very different view:

> I think because my wife became single when her son was an infant, she feels overly protective of him, and tries to protect him from life's difficulties. And her daughter is very timid and hides in her room a lot of the time, so there is not much of a relationship between me and her. Her daughter also ignores my son and essentially doesn't acknowledge his presence. This leads to a sort of tense atmosphere in the house.

Such statements reveal how issues between couples in stepfamilies are often played out through their children. Another husband put it even more succinctly, stating the following:

> . . . we tend to think that the other is picking on the other's children. The biggest problem reoccurring is this feeling of favoritism and perhaps jealousy . . . sometimes saying, "you are always favoring your children" . . . and "you are always babying them." Once we get angry with each other we are always pulling our children into it. That's the biggest problem we have.

In our research, we sought to examine how remarried couples cope with the interpersonal stressors that threaten stepfamily well-being. However, instead of considering the intraindividual results of coping, we were interested in examining how the coping strategies of one member of the couple might affect the quality of the relationship between the parents' spouse and the children in the family over the long-term. As we expected these effects to vary depending on the type of relationship (step vs. nonstep), we used the term *stepgap* to identify differences that emerge in the quality of the relationship between a parent and his or her children from a previous union and his or her relationship with stepchildren (DeLongis & Preece, 2002; Preece, 2000).

The Stepmother–Stepchild Relationship

Little research has examined the stepmother–stepchild relationship, probably because of the traditionally lower occurrence of stepmothers residing with their stepchildren. As recently as 20 years ago, 90% of mothers retained sole custody of children in a divorce (Hobart, 1994). However, in recent years, more men are seeking custody of their children, joint custody arrangements have become common, and the number of children residing with stepmothers, at least part of the time, has therefore increased.

In general, stepmothers tend to experience a great deal more stress, anxiety, depression, and anger about their role in the family than do mothers in other family structures (Santrock & Sitterle, 1987). Hobart (1994) proposed a number of explanations for why stepmothers more often have relationship problems with stepchildren than do stepfathers. For example, many husbands view the caring for and entertaining of children as their wives' responsibility. Both visiting and live-in stepchildren increase the housework load: There is more cooking, cleaning, shopping, and laundry, for example. In many households, this extra burden is largely on the wife's shoulders. Ambert (1989) found that husbands generally do not increase their level of help in the house when their children are visiting. In addition to the domestic responsibilities, some stepmothers find themselves having to cope with their husband's teenage children acting out in reaction to family disruptions. One stepmother explained her dilemma this way:

> My husband expects me to replace his ex-wife's role and take total responsibility for the stepchildren. I have to deal with the oldest stepchild's problems, and her relationship with the rest of the family. When I came into the relationship she was badly hurt from what had happened. Her mom left her when she was three years old and hasn't had anything to do with her since. When I moved in with my husband I think she felt a bond with him and I kind of took all the attention away when we were starting out. So there has always been a problem with that triangle. My stepdaughter has had emotional problems, and my husband and I have argued over how to deal with her problems because they have affected the whole family. It came to a real breaking point, and we ended up taking a parenting course that really helped us. I think I'm just starting to accept the whole thing now, and it has been six years. It's only in the last year or so that I've been able to accept responsibility for the two stepkids. I still have really bad feelings towards my husband's ex. I felt that she left her responsibilities. I also still feel the ghost of her around.

Shortly after the interview, the eldest stepdaughter discussed above moved away to live with her grandmother. However, then the younger stepdaughter began acting out and became difficult to deal with.

Further, visiting stepchildren may become involved in conflicts with the wife's children. If a mother intervenes, the stepchildren may perceive her as taking sides with her children against them (Ahrons & Wallisch, 1987). Because of the way men and women are socialized in our society, mothers usually care more and are more upset by these conflicts than are fathers (Hobart, 1994). In addition, to counteract guilty feelings about the divorce, a father may be more solicitous or extravagant with his children when they visit and be unwilling to use any form of discipline (Ambert, 1989). The wife may see this as favoritism and an indication that her husband cares more about his children than about her or her children. One stepmother described a situation involving her son (a teenager), husband, and her young stepson who was then living with them. She understood it this way:

> It's his first and only time as a parent. He's overdoing the parenting thing; he's more caring and sensitive with his child than with anyone else; and he expects me to back him up. He wasn't the residential parent of this child until a few years ago, and now he needs to do it right and wants to be totally involved.

At a follow-up interview 2 years later, the boy had decided to go back to live with his mother, and both partners were trying to cope with their sense of grief and impending loss.

Another explanation involves the differences in loyalty feelings children have for their mothers and for their fathers. For the father's children, their mother is usually the primary parent, and their feelings of loyalty to her are typically very strong. The child may resist closeness with the stepmother to avoid feelings of disloyalty toward his or her own mother. On the other hand, when children live with their mother and stepfather, loyalty feelings of children are less likely to interfere, as noncustodial fathers are often less involved with their children than are noncustodial mothers (Brooks, 1985, as cited in Hobart, 1994).

Stepmothers often make a tremendous effort to competently fulfill their role as a parent to their husbands' children. Remarried fathers and their new wives generally reported equal involvement and responsibility in their roles as parents (Clingempeel, Brand, & Ievoli, 1984). Nonetheless, children in these stepmother families perceived their stepmothers to be less involved with them than were their own fathers. These results suggest a dynamic in stepmother families in which stepmothers take responsibility for a goodly amount of the daily parenting activities but may not feel that they receive adequate recognition for their efforts, either from their husbands (Ambert, 1989) or from their stepchildren (Clingempeel et al., 1984). In families in which husbands are aware of such dynamics and attempt to cope with their wives' concerns in a positive and proactive manner, wives may find it easier to maintain a positive relationship with their husbands' children. One husband viewed his wife's concerns about her relationship with her stepson this way:

> Overall she really likes him and when she goes out of her way for him, she feels badly if he doesn't appreciate it or thank her. He's the only one in the household who isn't her biological child, and therefore she's more acutely aware of his responses. They both have strong personalities and he just battles back, because he's not that mature yet. My wife makes it worse because she notices little things and gets very sensitive, taking it all very personally, and she tends to brood about it. I don't want her to let him get away with unacceptable behavior, but I think it would be easier if she tried to ignore his behavior when it is just normal teenage stuff.

The Remarried Parent–Child Relationship

The quality of the parent–child relationship is negatively impacted by divorce and may not improve with remarriage. However, the effect of divorce on parent–child relationships may be different for sons and daughters and appears to depend partly on the gender of the parent. In a prospective study of divorce and remarriage, divorce appeared to result in less closeness between sons and mothers 12 years later (Booth & Amato, 1994). One stepmother in our study described her stepson's relationship with his mother this way:

> At first he always went to his mother's on the weekends and almost every day after school. She had remarried, but then a couple of years ago she had a baby and now he won't go over there any more, not even for his official visiting time every second weekend. He doesn't talk at all; he is very evasive; and when I had talks with him and asked him if he is happy living with us or if he would prefer to move back with his mom, he says that if he wanted to live with his mom he would have already gone.

However, no differences in closeness have been found for daughters and their divorced mothers as compared to daughters and mothers from intact marriages. Divorce appears to have a stronger negative impact on closeness with fathers for daughters than sons. A meta-analysis examining the effects of divorce on parent–child relationships concluded that parental divorce was significantly associated with poorer relationships with both parents, although the mean effect size was stronger for fathers than for mothers (Amato & Keith, 1991). In our study we found support for these conclusions, with many fathers showing declines across time in their closeness with their children. In one of the families in our study, the father gave up his relationship with his children from a previous relationship entirely to maintain peace in his new family. At the first interview, the father was still quite involved with his children but the brewing problems were apparent from his new wife's description:

> His family (his kids, his parents, his ex-wife) refuses to accept me as the children's stepmother. I am not invited or included for any family occasions. My husband won't confront his family, and continues to make plans for social events that exclude me. He just says that I would not get along with his ex-wife and his mother. He's very afraid of conflict and will do anything to avoid it. If someone is rude to me, he says he didn't hear it. Then he doesn't deal with it because it never happened. His wife is influencing the kids to relate to their dad as if I don't exist. She will not go along with them having a relationship with their dad and me in our own home.

In this family, the father was put in a position in which he felt he had to choose between his wife and his children. He chose his wife, and at the next interview, two years later, his wife stated that they had "given up on trying to blend" and that this had reduced the stress on their relationship significantly. However, he had absolutely no contact with his children from the previous marriage. As he put it, "I don't call them, and they don't call me."

Remarried custodial fathers often report being more actively involved in parenting their children than fathers from intact families, but remarried custodial mothers still report being much more involved in discipline, observation of their children's recreational activities, and provision of comfort and sympathy than do remarried custodial fathers (Clingempeel et al., 1984). However, adolescents in divorced families and in stepfamilies have also been shown to experience the highest levels of mother–adolescent disagreements and the lowest levels of supervision (Demo & Acock, 1996).

Parent–Child Relationship Quality in Our Sample of Stepfamilies

In our study, both husbands and wives reported feeling closer to their own children than to their stepchildren (DeLongis & Preece, 2002). However, wives generally reported having greater closeness and less tension in their relationships with their children than their husbands did with their children. Further, wives experienced more tension with their stepchildren than husbands did with their stepchildren. In terms of changes over time, husbands reported a decrease in closeness and an increase in tension with their own children over a 2-year period.

In order to understand better some of the changes in relationship quality that are confounded with adolescence, we examined changes in relationship quality separately for children of different ages (Preece, 2000). For children between 12 and 17 years of age at the beginning of the study, the amount of tension in the relationship reported by parents was the highest of all age groups. However, 2 years later, tension with children in this group had decreased substantially, suggesting that most stepfamilies are able to cope successfully with tension in the parent–child relationships with adolescent children and that the quality of the relationship does improve substantially, with average levels of tension 2 years later reduced to a level similar to that of preadolescent children.

Daily Coping in Stepfamilies

Two broad functions of coping have generally been emphasized in the stress and coping literature: problem focused and emotion focused (Lazarus & Folkman, 1984). Problem-focused coping involves attempts to change the person–environment relation directly, whereas emotion-focused coping is geared toward managing negative emotions generated by the stressful situation. When coping with stressors that are primarily interpersonal, however, an additional function is required. Within the family, where the development and maintenance of good relationships is paramount to well-being, forms of coping that focus on repairing, improving, or preserving one's relationships with others become critical. Relationship-focused coping has therefore been proposed as a third function of coping (Coyne & Smith, 1991; DeLongis & O'Brien, 1990; O'Brien & DeLongis, 1997).

Another important issue in studying coping with interpersonal stressors is obtaining data that are recorded soon after the actual stressor. Retrospective bias can quickly contaminate accurate reporting. We therefore used a daily record methodology to examine the stressful issues facing parents in stepfamilies. Parents were asked to report daily on the strategies they used to cope with family stress and how the day-to-day quality of their relationships was affected. Coping strategies were measured with the Brief Ways of Coping (BWOC) developed for use in daily process studies (DeLongis & Preece, 2002; see also Folkman, Lazarus, Dunkel-Schetter, DeLongis, & Gruen, 1986; Newth & DeLongis, 2004; Preece, 2000). The scale measures problem-focused, emotion-focused, and relationship-focused coping strategies.

In this chapter, we focus on those coping strategies that we consider dyadic coping strategies. These strategies have an *other* focus and are likely to affect not only the stressor and the coper but also other family members involved in the stressful event. Each of the five strategies that we believe are relevant to the investigation of relationship-focused coping is described next.

Empathic Coping

Empathic coping refers to attempts to perceive the emotional experience of others involved in the situation. A particularly important function of empathic coping is its ability to facilitate positive interactions between individuals under stressful circumstances. Empathy is more likely to be used in situations in which a loved one's well-being is at stake (Preece, 1996).

Support Provision

Support provision involves efforts to express caring or understanding in a non-judgmental way. Although only the *seeking* of emotional support has traditionally been thought of as a coping strategy, we would argue that *providing* support can also be an effective way of coping with a stressor involving a loved one. We have found that providing support is most likely in situations in which individuals feel they have some control over the situation and a loved one's well-being is threatened.

Compromise

Surprisingly little research has focused on the construct of compromise. However, there are a number of similar constructs that are relevant. For example, a theory of accommodation processes has been advanced that bears some resemblance to the construct of compromise. Accommodation has been defined as an individual's willingness to engage in a constructive reaction given a partner's potentially destructive behavior (Rusbult, Verette, Whitney, Slovik, & Lipkus, 1991). The decision to accommodate tends to be associated with features of the relationship. In particular, individuals are more likely to accommodate in relationships in which they have a high level of commitment. It has also been proposed that there might be a social cost to the decision to accommodate. In a healthy relationship, for example, a fair degree of mutuality in the process of accommodation is expected. However, if one partner carries most of the accommodative burden in the relationship, he or she will probably experience some personal distress as a consequence (see also DeLongis, Bolger, & Kessler, 1987). This may be a particular hazard in step-families in which parents are making extensive efforts to accommodate to the needs and wishes of a number of children, ex-partners, and extended family on both sides.

One of the most important determinants of an individual's decision to cooperate may be the expectation of reciprocity. Individuals are usually more cooperative when they expect that others will also cooperate. The idea of reci-procity is at the heart of all stable relationships and is a basic norm in all social interactions (Thibaut & Kelley, 1959). A study of husbands and wives coping with daily marital tension (DeLongis et al., 1987) found that although wives' use of compromise did not reduce the amount of distress they experi-enced, it was related to a decrease in the amount of distress reported by their husbands. This suggests that compromise in an intimate relationship may benefit primarily the other partner and perhaps the relationship but carries no immediate benefits to the self.

Our own stepfamily data indicate that use of compromise is greater when stressors are appraised as a threat to the coper's well-being. Specifically, such stressors were appraised as involving either the threat of "losing someone's respect or love" or "not getting the support and understanding you want." This suggests that willingness to compromise may often be motivated by the need to preserve one's place in a relationship. However, participants were more likely to use compromise when they appraised themselves as having a fair amount of control over how the situation was handled.

Confrontation

Competitive and dominating behaviors such as confrontation are more likely to be used to deal with interpersonal conflict when the individual's concern is focused primarily on his or her own goals rather than on the needs of the other (Rahim, 1983). Our results suggest that confrontation is most likely to be used when individuals appraise themselves as having significant control over the situation. Confronted individuals may concede in the short term, but the like-lihood of future cooperation may be reduced as a result of the negative emotions, such as resentment, anger, hurt, and sadness, they may experience. Equally problematic, the confronter is likely to be encouraged by the conces-sion to continue to employ similar strategies in the future. Over time, such interaction patterns may lead to the escalation of hostile and aggressive behaviors (Patterson, 1982). In our sample of stepfamilies, wives reported using confrontation to cope with family stressors significantly more often than did their husbands.

Interpersonal Withdrawal

We operationalized interpersonal withdrawal as coping that has a punitive and negative tone and includes such behaviors as withdrawing from the person involved, giving them the "silent treatment," sulking, and making efforts to "keep my feelings to myself" and to "keep others from knowing about the problem or my feelings." When participants felt that their position in an important relationship was threatened and they perceived themselves as having little control, they reported a greater tendency to withdraw from the person involved or otherwise try to avoid the problem. Wives also reported using interpersonal withdrawal to cope with family stressors significantly more than did their husbands.

Stressor Type as a Predictor of Coping

The two most common sources of family stress that emerged in this sample were marital conflict and child misbehavior. This was consistent with previous findings from research on both families and stepfamilies (Kheshgi-Genovese & Genovese, 1997). Consistent with our previous research on married couples (Folkman, Lazarus, Gruen, & DeLongis, 1986), we found that our respondents coped differently depending on the stressor, an indication that contextual factors played a significant and independent role in coping.

When coping with marital conflict, as compared to child misbehavior, respondents reported using more empathic coping, support provision, compromise, interpersonal withdrawal, and less confrontation (Lee-Baggley, Preece, & DeLongis, 2004). Both husbands and wives were more likely to take an egalitarian perspective by trying to see their spouse's perspective, offering support, compromising and acknowledging their own contributions to the conflict. They were also more likely to report withdrawing in response to marital conflict than to child misbehavior; they were less likely to try to understand their child's point of view and more likely to confront the child about the behavior. Withdrawal in response to child misbehavior may be a less appropriate response given the responsibility of the parenting role.

The Effect of Daily Coping on Parent–Child Relationship Quality

LAGGED EFFECTS OF DAILY COPING. We previously found that most stressors have an immediate effect on mood but that emotional habituation occurs by the second day for all stressors except interpersonal conflicts (Bolger, DeLongis, Kessler, & Schilling, 1989). The longer lasting effects of interpersonal conflict have been found to have a physiological component as well. For example, in a study of newly married couples, negative conflict had immunosuppressive effects that persisted for at least the following day (Kiecolt-Glaser et al., 1993). By using a 24-hour lag, researchers avoid contamination of relationship quality reports by negative mood from other stressful events and strengthen causal inference regarding the effect of coping on relationship quality. For the analyses that examine coping as a predictor of changes in relationship quality, we used the average amount of coping reported by parents across 7 days as a contextual variable, (i.e., controlling for the general interpersonal climate while isolating the day-to-day effects of coping on next-day relationship quality. In contrast, when we examined whether relationship quality predicts changes in coping, *average* relationship quality across the 7 days was used as the contextual variable.

COPING AS A PREDICTOR OF NEXT-DAY PARENT–CHILD RELATIONSHIP QUALITY. The results of the analyses of across-day relations between coping and relationship quality between parents and children in stepfamilies indicated that a clear connection could be established and that fluctuations in daily relationship quality could be considered outcomes of coping. For example, after controlling for parents' average use of compromise as well as parents' reports of affection from their own children on the same day, we found that greater use of compromise on one day was related to an increase in affection and support from parents' own children on the next day, but not from stepchildren. For these analyses, we used a matched design, with stepchildren and own children nested within families. This method allowed us to draw strong conclusions, and by using an indicator variable to represent the stepgap, we were able to compare statistically the effect of each parent's coping on relationship quality for both stepchildren and own children. Further, as the distinction between children is reversed for the other parent, characteristics of the children are perfectly controlled.

The results suggest that parents' own children tend to reward their parents with increased affection for using compromise when dealing with family stressors. Such lagged responses may be entirely outside of awareness, reflecting deeply ingrained patterns of parent–child interactions. Interactions early in childhood may lay down memory traces that are activated by current interpersonal situations (Sullivan, 1953) and determine behavior in those situations (Carson, 1991). No such pattern was discerned for parents and their stepchildren. Relations between stepchildren and stepparents do not have the same history and may therefore be more deliberate. A comment by a study participant emphasized the self-consciousness a stepparent may feel when establishing a relationship with stepchildren. This stepmother, who became an *instant* mother when her husbands' young children moved into their home, stated the following:

> I have lost my freedom and my privacy. There are moments of considerable resentment on my part that of course I must bring to my relationship with them. I don't have the natural bond that's felt with a birth parent and the children. So it's an ongoing effort to extend myself in that way.

Interpersonal withdrawal was also related to changes in relationship quality, but only for stepchildren. That is, increased use of interpersonal withdrawal was related to a significant decrease in tension with stepchildren on the following day. These results suggest that stepparents are also reinforced for their behavior, but in this case, for their use of interpersonal withdrawal. Interpersonal withdrawal by stepparents was related to a decrease in tension with stepchildren on the following day. Parents' use of interpersonal withdrawal as a way of avoiding tension with stepchildren may quickly become a self-sustaining and ultimately detrimental behavior.

PARENT–CHILD RELATIONSHIP QUALITY AS A PREDICTOR OF NEXT-DAY COPING. Tension with either their own children or their stepchildren did not predict parents' coping on the following day. Stepchildren's demonstrations of affection and support predicted a reduction in stepparents' use of compromise the following day (as compared to their average levels). This unexpected result suggests that stepparents may not think to reward their stepchild's prosocial behavior; instead they interpret such behavior as an opportunity to gain control in a generally out-of-control situation. Unfortunately, such a response is likely to quickly extinguish any future attempts on the part of stepchildren to develop emotional closeness with the stepparent. The results presented here are consistent with general observations that relationships and conflict interactions reciprocally reframe each other (Canary, Cupach, & Messman, 1995).

Use of confrontation, on the other hand, did not have lagged relations with relationship quality in either direction. Some researchers have indicated that anger is not nearly as corrosive to relationships as is withdrawal (Gottman & Levenson, 1992). Further, conflict can have a positive role in the development of a relationship (Canary et al., 1995). It is not always clear empirically whether conflict is a symptom of relationship difficulties or a sign that active effort is being put forth to develop an alliance. In fact, contrary to expectations, neither interpersonal withdrawal nor confrontation has a particularly negative impact on relationship quality at a single time point. However, as a habitual form of response to interpersonal conflict, confrontation may become problematic because of the reactions it elicits in others. For example, parents who reported greater typical use of confrontation also reported higher daily levels of tension with their own children.

Although confronted individuals may concede defeat in the short term, the likelihood of future cooperation may be reduced as a result of the resentment they experience. An immediate short-term success may provide reinforcement to the confronter, thus encouraging continued use of similar strategies. Over time, however, such interaction patterns may lead to the escalation of hostile and aggressive behaviors (Patterson, 1983).

Parents' Typical Ways of Coping as Predictors of Changes in Parent–Child Relationship Quality Over Time

Parental behavior has been shown to be highly stable across time (Holden & Miller, 1999). Therefore, it is reasonable to assume that small effects of parental behavior across days are likely to become larger effects across years. Further, research on stress and coping has shown that coping behavior, although situation specific, is also quite stable over time (Carver, Scheier, & Weintraub, 1989; Endler & Parker, 1990). We examined parents' typical ways of coping over a 7-day period and used them to predict their partner's relationship quality with children in the stepfamily 2 years later. Our results indicate that daily family responses to interpersonal stressors have cumulative effects on parent–child relationships over time (DeLongis & Preece, 2002).

Wives' use of confrontation to cope with family stressors had a negative effect on their husbands' relationships with their stepchildren. Specifically, wives' greater use of confrontation, controlling for their husbands' closeness to the stepchildren at Time 1, predicted decreased closeness between their husbands' and the wives' own children at Time 2. On the other hand, lower levels of daily confrontation used by wives predicted increased closeness between husbands and their stepchildren at Time 2. This result suggests a dynamic that may be involved in promoting the disengaged parenting style typical of stepfathers (Hetherington, 1993). In a conflictual family atmosphere, husbands may be even more inclined to avoid involvement with their stepchildren.

Wives' relationships with their own children were affected by husbands' coping. In particular, the results suggested that when husbands withdraw, it may negatively impact wives' relationships with their own children. Wives whose husbands reported higher levels of withdrawal also reported an increase in tension with their own children two years later. One mother described how her husband was negatively affecting her relationship with her daughter. "My teenaged daughter is pregnant, and I want to be there for her, but my husband gets really jealous. He is suffocating me, and I need to be available to my daughter. She needs me right now."

Husbands who withdraw consistently in response to family stress may be individuals who do not cope well with any kind of stress. Their lack of proactive coping strategies may preclude the development of a cohesive stepfamily unit because of either their unwillingness or inability to extend themselves in an effortful way. Alternatively, husbands who withdraw consistently may be reacting to the unexpected complexities of stepfamily life. If their first efforts at coping are not successful, they may begin to withdraw increasingly as the most effective way to avoid family tension. Unfortunately, the results presented here also suggest that wives cannot hope to grow closer to their stepchildren and maintain good relations with their own children without their husbands' active participation in daily life.

Together, these results suggest that in stepfamilies in which wives report using higher amounts of confrontation to cope with family stressors, husbands may withdraw. The result tends to be a decrease in husbands' closeness with stepchildren over time. Further, in stepfamilies in which husbands reported more interpersonal withdrawal to cope with family stressors, their wives reported a decrease in closeness with their stepchildren and greater tension with their own children two year later. Wives' use of interpersonal withdrawal was also related to lower closeness with their own children two years later, although the negative impact on wives' stepchildren was negligible.

Considering Context

Our examination of stress and coping processes and their effects on relationship quality have consistently demonstrated that a consideration of context adds a great deal to our predictive models. In general, we found that the results of within-day analyses more often demonstrated the immediate effects of stressors, whereas analyses of lagged effects demonstrated the role that relationship characteristics play in determining the longer lasting effects of stressful situations. In addition, our results show clearly that the quality of interpersonal relationships both affect and are affected by stress and coping processes.

These results warn against considering only individual outcomes when studying the relations among stress, coping, and well-being. When stress and coping processes are considered in a social vacuum, we may unwittingly create the illusion that people generally adapt to stress in an autonomous, solitary fashion. Consequently, we may be more likely to view adaptational problems as being primarily attributable to personality vulnerabilities, faulty perceptions, or insufficient personal initiative. Our research shows that coping does not arise solely from the individual's own efforts but can be powerfully affected by marital partners, families, and other social units. Our understanding of the processes involved in coping with stress will be hampered if we view individuals in isolation, apart from their significant social contexts. Indeed, individualistic notions of stress adaptation are of limited use in describing and explaining family patterns of adaptation that operate in a more systemic, interdependent manner. Even more importantly, an individualistic focus may obscure our understanding of the psychosocial processes that are central to managing stress in interpersonal contexts. Our results therefore emphasize the importance of considering psychosocial processes in the development of interventions designed to improve ways of coping with interpersonal stressors.

Methodology for Studying Stepfamilies

The study of stepfamilies is fraught with complexities that present methodological problems for researchers. Because of the many variants of stepfamily composition, there is often confusion about what types of stepfamilies are being studied. In many stepfamilies, not all family members necessarily reside full time in one household. In one stepfamily household there may be several combinations of full- and part-time living arrangements for different children. Some researchers have attempted to develop typologies to describe different types of stepfamilies (e.g., Clingempeel, Brand, & Segal, 1987; Wald, 1981). These typologies describe from 9 to 15 variations of stepfamilies but still do not account for the additional complexities that occur when remarried couples have children from the current union. Findings from research on stepfamilies are difficult to generalize, as many studies have focused on only one member of the remarried family, collapsed data across different structural types of stepfamilies, and failed to control for a number of other variables related to outcomes. Further, for studies that compare means across groups, it is often difficult to obtain the necessary number of participants for each category, let alone try to match across groups for such characteristics as socioeconomic status, age, presence of stepsiblings, or children from the new marriage.

Such difficulties have forced researchers to take a more eclectic and flexible view of stepfamilies. Instead of focusing on differences between family structures, it may be more profitable to identify variables that reliably predict differences in important outcomes and use a multivariate approach. In this research, the characterization of families as complex groups leads to the application of multilevel modeling as a statistical technique for the analysis of data with a hierarchical nesting structure. In the case of families, children can be considered as nested within the parental structure (Snijders & Bosker, 1999). All children in the family have the same parents (or stepparents), so their relationship outcomes are not independent.

There are a number of distinct advantages to the use of multilevel models to analyze this type of data. First, simpler methods, such as ordinary least squares regression analysis, do not take into account the grouping of data in families, and therefore, the models are misspecified and the results unreliable. A second advantage of multilevel models is that the observed variance is decomposed into variance because of differences between children and variance because of differences between families so that explanatory variables can be modeled separately. A third advantage is that this method of analysis considers variance in the slopes separately from variance at either level. A fourth advantage is that in multilevel analyses, it is possible to compare relationship quality of stepchildren and biological children to the same parent initially using data from those families that contain both types of children but *borrowing strength* through an iterative process from those families that are missing data (in this case, children). In other words, for those families in which only the wives' children are described, the data they provide are still considered in the calculation of the final coefficients even though they cannot provide within-family information on the stepgap.

This type of analysis is also useful for the examination of daily diary data (DeLongis, Hemphill, & Lehman, 1992). Our approach is to consider days as nested within individuals (husbands and wives). In turn, these individuals are nested within families. For some of the diary data analyses, a three-level model was used. One of the advantages of such a model is that it allows for the generalization of results to the within-family case. Another approach was used to focus on within-couple relationships. For these analyses, a two-level model containing days for each couple nested within families was used. When complex data such as ours are aggregated, relations between macrolevels cannot be used to make assertions about microlevel relations. However, with multilevel analyses, we were able to examine microlevel relations as well as how these microlevel relations varied depending on macrolevel variables.

References

Ahrons, C. R., & Wallisch, L. (1987). Parenting in the binuclear family: Relationship between biological and stepparents. In K. Pasley & M. Ihinger-Tallman (Eds.), *Remarriage and stepparenting: Current research and theory* (pp. 225–256). New York: Guilford Press.

Amato, R., & Keith, B. (1991). Consequence of parental divorce for children's well-being: A meta-analysis. *Psychological Bulletin, 110,* 26–46.

Ambert, A. (1989) *Ex-spouses and new spouses: A study of relationships.* Greenwich, CT: JAI Press.

Bolger, N., DeLongis, A., Kessler, R. C., & Schilling, E. A. (1989). The emotional effects of daily stress. *Journal of Personality and Social Psychology, 57,* 808–818.

Booth, A., & Amato, P. R. (1994). Parent marital quality, parental divorce, and relations with parents. *Journal of Marriage and the Family, 56,* 21–34.

Bray, J. H. (1991). Psychosocial factors affecting custodial and visitation arrangements. *Behavioral Sciences and the Law, 9,* 419–437.

Bray, J. H., & Berger, S. H. (1993). Development issues in stepfamilies research project: Family relationships and parent–child interactions. *Journal of Family Psychology, 7,* 76–90.

Bray, J. H., & Hetherington, E. M. (1993). Families in transition: Introduction and overview. *Journal of Family Psychology, 7,* 3–8.

Brooks, A. (1985, January 13). Stepchildren on panel tell parents how it is. *The New York Times,* B5

Canary, D. J., Cupach, W. R., & Messman, S. J. (1995). *Relationship conflict*. Thousand Oaks, CA: Sage.

Carson, R. C. (1991). The social-interaction viewpoint. In M. Hersen, A. E. Kazdin, & A. S. Bellack (Eds.), *The clinical psychology handbook* (2nd ed.). New York: Pergamon Press.

Carver, C. S., Scheier, M. F., & Weintraub, J. K. (1989). Assessing coping strategies: A theoretically based approach. *Journal of Personality and Social Psychology, 61*, 404–412.

Clingempeel, W. G., Brand, E., & Ievoli, R. (1984). Stepparent–stepchild relationships in stepmother and stepfather families: A multi-method study. *Family Relations, 33*, 465–473.

Clingempeel, W. G., Brand, E., & Segal, S. (1987). A multilevel-multivariable-developmental perspective for future research on stepfamilies. In K. Pasley & M. Ihinger-Tallman (Eds.), *Remarriage and stepparenting: Current research and theory* (pp. 65–93). New York: Guilford Press.

Coleman, M., & Ganong, L. (1990). Remarriage and stepfamily research in the 80s: New interest in an old family form. *Journal of Marriage and the Family, 52*, 925–940.

Coyne, J. C., & Smith, D. A. F. (1991). Couples coping with myocardial infarction: I. A contextual perspective on wives' distress. *Journal of Personality and Social Psychology, 6*, 404–412.

Cramer, D. (1985). Psychological adjustment and the facilitative nature of close relationships. *British Journal of Medical Psychology, 58*, 165–168.

Crosbie-Burnett, M. (1984). The centrality of the step relationship: A challenge to family theory and practice. *Family Relations, 33*, 459–464.

Crosbie-Burnett, M. (1989). Application of family stress theory to remarriage: A model for assessing and helping stepfamilies. *Family Relations, 38*, 323–331.

Crosbie-Burnett, M., & Ahrons, C. R. (1985). From divorce to remarriage: Implications for therapy with families in transition. *Journal of Psychotherapy and the Family, 1*, 121–137.

DeLongis, A., Bolger, N., & Kessler, R. C. (1987, August). *Coping with marital conflict*. Paper presented at the meeting of the American Psychological Association, New York.

DeLongis, A., Hemphill, K. J., & Lehman, D. R. (1992). A structured diary methodology for the study of daily events. In F. B. Bryant, J. Edwards, L. Heath, E. J. Posanac, & R. S. Tinsdale (Eds.), *Methodological issues in applied social psychology* (pp. 83–109). New York: Plenum Press.

DeLongis, A., & O'Brien, T. B. (1990). An interpersonal framework for stress and coping: An application to the families of Alzheimer's patients. In M. A. P. Stephens, J. H. Crowther, S. E. Hobfoll, & D. L. Tennenbaum (Eds.), *Stress and coping in later-life families* (pp. 221–238). Washington, DC: Hemisphere Publication Services.

DeLongis, A., & Preece, M. (2002). Emotional and relational consequences of coping in stepfamilies. [Special issue on Emotions and the Family]. *Marriage and Family Review, 34*, 115–138.

Demo, D. H., & Acock, A. C. (1996). Family structure, family process, and adolescent well-being. *Journal of Research on Adolescence, 6*, 457–488.

Endler, N. S., & Parker, J. D. A. (1990). Multidimensional assessment of coping: A critical evaluation. *Journal of Personality and Social Psychology, 58*, 844–854.

Feldman, S. I., Downey, G., & Schaffer-Neitz, R. (1999). Pain, negative mood, and perceived support in chronic pain patients: A daily diary study of people with reflex sympathetic dystrophy syndrome. *Journal of Consulting and Clinical Psychology, 67*, 776–785.

Fishman, B. (1983). The economic behavior of stepfamilies. *Family Relations, 32*, 359–366.

Folkman, S., Lazarus, R. S., Dunkel-Schetter, C., DeLongis, A., & Gruen, R. J. (1986). Dynamics of a stressful encounter: Cognitive appraisal, coping, and encounter outcomes. *Journal of Personality and Social Psychology, 50*, 992–1003.

Folkman, S., Lazarus, R. S., Gruen, R., & DeLongis, A. (1986). Appraisal, coping, health status, and psychological symptoms. *Journal of Personality and Social Psychology, 50*, 571–579.

Ganong, L. H., & Coleman, M. (1994). *Remarried family relationships*. Thousand Oaks, CA: Sage.

Gottman, J. M., & Levenson, R. W. (1992). Marital processes predictive of later dissolution: Behavior, physiology, and health. *Journal of Personality and Social Psychology, 63*, 221–233.

Hetherington, E. M. (1982). Effects of divorce on parents and children. In M. Lamb (Ed.), *Nontraditional families: Parenting and child development*, Hillsdale, NJ: Erlbaum.

Hetherington, E. M. (1993). An overview of the Virginia Longitudinal Study of Divorce and Remarriage with a focus on early adolescence. *Journal of Family Psychology, 7*, 39–56.

Hetherington, E. M., Bridges, M., & Insabella, G. M. (1998). What matters? What does not? Five perspectives on the association between marital transitions and children's adjustment. *American Psychologist, 53*, 167–184.

Hetherington, E. M., & Jodl, K. M. (1994). Stepfamilies as settings for child development. In A. Booth & J. Dunn (Eds.), *Stepfamilies: Who benefits? Who does not?* Hillsdale, NJ: Erlbaum.

Hobart, C. (1990). Experiences of remarried families. *Journal of Divorce, 13,* 121–144.

Hobart, C. (1991). Conflict in remarriages. *Journal of Divorce and Remarriage, 15,* 69–86.

Hobart, C. (1994). New relationships: Remarriage and stepparent. In L. E. Larson, J. Walter Goltz, & C. W. Hobart (Eds.), *Families in Canada: Social context, continuities, and changes.* Scarborough, Ontario, Canada: Prentice Hall.

Holden, G. W., & Miller, P. C. (1999). Enduring and different: A meta-analysis of the similarity in parents' child rearing. *Psychological Bulletin, 125,* 223–254.

Jacobson, D. (1990). Stress and support in stepfamily formation: The cultural context of social support. In B. R. Sarason, I. G. Sarason, & G. R. Pierce (Eds.), *Social support: An interactional view* (pp. 199–218). New York: Wiley

Kheshgi-Genovese, Z., & Genovese, T. A. (1997). Developing the spousal relationship within stepfamilies. *Families in Society: The Journal of Contemporary Human Services, 78,* 255–264.

Kiecolt-Glaser, J. K., Malarkey, W. B., Chee, M. A., Newton, T., Cacioppo, J. T., Mao, H. Y., & Glaser, R. (1993). Negative behavior during marital conflict is associated with immunological down-regulation. *Psychosomatic Medicine, 55,* 395–409.

Kramer, B. J. (1993). Expanding the conceptualization of caregiver coping: The importance of relationship-focused coping strategies. *Family Relations, 42,* 383–391.

Lazarus, R. S., & Folkman, S. (1984). *Stress, appraisal, and coping.* New York: Springer Publishing Company.

Lee-Baggley, D., Preece, M., & DeLongis, A. (2004). *Coping in context: The role of personality and situation.* Manuscript submitted for publication.

McGoldrick, M., & Carter, B. (1988). Forming a remarried family. In B. Carter & M. McGoldrick (Eds.), *The changing family life cycle* (pp. 399–429). New York: Gardner Press.

Mills, D. (1984). A model for stepfamily development. *Family Relations, 33,* 365–372.

Newth, S., & DeLongis, A. (2004). Individual differences, mood and coping with chronic pain in rheumatoid arthritis: A daily process analysis. *Psychology and Health, 19,* 283–305.

O'Brien, T. B., & DeLongis, A. (1997). Coping with chronic stress: An interpersonal perspective. In B. H. Gottlieb (Ed.), *Coping with chronic stress* (pp. 161–190). New York: Plenum Press.

Papernow, P. L. (1987). Thickening the "middle ground": Dilemmas and vulnerabilities of remarried couples. *Psychotherapy, 24,* 630–639.

Patterson, G. R. (1982). *Coercive family process.* Eugene, OR: Castalia.

Patterson, G. R. (1983). Stress: A change agent for family process. In N. Garmezy & M. Rutter (Eds.), *Stress, coping, and development in children.* New York: McGraw-Hill.

Preece, M. (1996). *Coping with interpersonal stressors: Issues of love and status.* Unpublished master's thesis, University of British Columbia, Vancouver, Canada.

Preece, M. (2000). *Exploring the stepgap: How parents' ways of coping with daily family stressors impact stepparent–stepchild relationship quality in stepfamilies.* Unpublished doctoral dissertation, University of British Columbia, Vancouver, Canada.

Rahim, J. A. (1983). A measure of styles of handling interpersonal conflict. *Academy of Management Journal, 26,* 368–376.

Rusbult, C. E., Verette, J., Whitney, G. A., Slovik, L. F., & Lipkus, I. (1991). Accomodation processes in close relationships: Theory and preliminary empirical evidence. *Journal of Personality and Social Psychology, 60,* 53–78.

Santrock, J. W., & Sitterle, K. (1987). Parent–child relationships in stepmother families. In K. Pasley & M. Ihinger-Tallman (Eds.), *Remarriage and stepparenting today: Current research and theory* (pp. 273–299). New York: Guilford Press.

Snijders, T. B., & Bosker, R. J. (1999). *Multilevel analysis: An introduction to basic and advanced multilevel modeling.* London: Sage.

Sullivan, H. S. (1953). *The interpersonal theory of psychiatry.* New York: Norton.

Thibaut, J. W., & Kelly, H. H. (1959). *The social psychology of groups.* New York: Wiley.

Visher, E. B., & Visher, J. S. (1988). *Old loyalties, new ties: Therapeutic strategies with stepfamilies.* New York: Brunner/Mazel.

Wald, E. (1981). *The remarried family: Challenge and promise.* New York: Family Service Association of America.

Wallerstein, J. S., & Blakeslee, S. (1989). *Second chances: Men, women and children a decade after divorce.* New York: Ticknor & Fields.

White, L. K., & Booth, A. (1985). The quality and stability of remarriages: The role of stepchildren. *American Sociological Review, 50,* 689–698.

Zeppa, A., & Norem, R. H. (1993). Stressors, manifestations of stress, and first family/stepfamily group membership. *Journal of Divorce and Remarriage, 19,* 3–24.

Zill, N., Morrison, D. R., & Coiro, M. J. (1993). Long-term effects of parental divorce on parent–child relationships, adjustment, and achievement in young adulthood. *Journal of Family Psychology, 7,* 91–103.

Part II

Social Support, Dyadic Coping, and Interpersonal Communication

4

The Relationship Enhancement Model of Social Support

Carolyn E. Cutrona, Daniel W. Russell, and Kelli A. Gardner

When faced with disappointment, loss, or overwhelming challenge, people attach great importance to the behavior of their intimate partner. Times of duress provide a *test* of whether the partner can be relied on to offer comfort, advice, encouragement, and assistance, the key elements of social support. In this chapter, we argue that whether support is provided has profound implications for relationship quality, stability, and the health of both partners. We propose a new model of the link between social support and health, the *relationship enhancement model*. The relationship enhancement model states that when certain conditions are met, social support from an intimate partner builds trust and the belief that the partner is motivated by genuine concern for one's well-being and will provide care when needed. Trust is a critical component of relationship quality and stability. Both the quality and stability of intimate relationships are, in turn, tied to mental and physical health outcomes. Thus, social support affects health outcomes through its influence on the quality and stability of intimate relationships.

The relationship enhancement model departs from existing models of social support and health in several ways. First, the model proposes that social support's most important contribution to health is through its impact on the quality of ongoing relationships. Supportive acts from an intimate partner during times of duress set in motion a series of emotional and cognitive events that strengthen the relationship and prevent health-damaging relationship conflict, deterioration, and dissolution. Second, the model views the effects of social support in a longer time frame than does previous models. The influence of social support is not limited to the days and weeks that surround specific stressful events. Rather, social support is viewed as influencing attitudes, emotions, and behaviors across the entire duration of an intimate relationship. Third, distinct roles are defined for social support behaviors and perceptions of social support. A set of conditions is described in which support-intended behaviors contribute to subjective evaluations of support availability. In the absence of these conditions, a supportive act will not lead to the perception of the provider as supportive. This is important because beliefs about the partner's supportiveness and motivation to provide support are central to the beneficial effects of social support on relationship quality and health.

Existing Models of Social Support's Effects on Health

Two previous models have been proposed to explain the benefits of social support. The *buffering hypothesis* focuses on support's ability to protect against the deleterious effects of negative life events on health and well-being (Cassel, 1976; Cobb, 1976; Cohen & Wills, 1985). In this model, supportive acts help stressed individuals to make less threatening appraisals of stressors, believe in their ability to cope effectively, and take constructive steps to eliminate stressors. Social support is viewed as a shield that diminishes the immediate impact of negative life events on health and well-being. A longer time frame is adopted in the relationship enhancement model. In addition to the immediate stress-reducing effects of partner support, consistent supportive responses from the partner have a long-term effect on relationship quality and stability. By preserving and enhancing relationship quality, social support decreases an important class of health-damaging stressors: the deterioration and dissolution of close relationships. A second traditional approach to understanding social support's effects on health, the *direct effects model*, posits that people benefit from social support both in the presence and absence of stressful life events. Integration into a supportive network confers ongoing benefits, including predictability, stability, clear role expectations, and a sense of belonging and purpose (Cobb, 1976; Weiss, 1974). The relationship enhancement model is similar to the direct effects model in that support is viewed as contributing to people's quality of daily life over an extended period of time. It differs from the direct effects model in its explicit focus on relationship quality and stability.

Overview of the Model

We briefly describe the relationship enhancement model of social support in intimate relationships and then provide a more detailed examination of each component of the model. Empirical support for hypothesized links between variables is presented when available. The model is shown in Figure 4.1.

The relationship enhancement process begins with individual supportive behaviors by the intimate partner. A crucial role is accorded to how the recip-

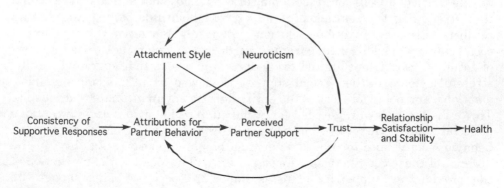

Figure 4.1.   The relationship enhancement model of social support.

ient of the support explains the causes or reasons that support was provided. These causal explanations are termed *attributions*. Partner support that is viewed as reflective of the partner's internal and enduring traits contributes to perceptions of the spouse as a reliable source of social support in times of need (Fincham & Bradbury, 1990). In other words, supportive behaviors from the partner only increase perceived social support if they are viewed as motivated by internal, stable traits, such as kindness, caring, or commitment to the relationship.

Consistency and internality of partner support are not the only variables that affect evaluations of perceived social support. Individual difference variables also influence both attributions for partner behavior and support evaluations. One individual difference variable that affects perceived support and attributions for partner behavior is adult attachment orientation. Individuals with a secure attachment orientation report higher perceived social support and make more benevolent attributions for their partner's behavior than those with an insecure attachment orientation (Gallo & Smith, 2001; Hazan & Shaver, 1987). A second individual difference variable that affects both attributions and perceived social support is neuroticism. Individuals who are high on neuroticism perceive lower levels of social support and make more negative attributions for partner behavior (Halamandaris & Power, 1999; Russell, Hessling, & Cutrona, 2000).

The next pathway in the proposed model leads from perceptions regarding partner support to trust. In this chapter, we have adopted the definition of trust proposed by Holmes and colleagues (Holmes & Rempel, 1989; Rempel, Holmes, & Zanna, 1985): the confident expectation that one's partner can be relied upon to care for one and be responsive to one's needs, now and in the future. When people perceive their partner as a reliable source of social support and believe that the support is a reflection of their partner's genuine caring, their level of trust grows. They come to expect that their partner will be responsive to their needs and strive to enhance their well-being long into the future.

Trust plays an important role in the relationship enhancement model because it is a determinant of relationship quality and stability. As we describe in more detail below, trust influences marital quality and stability through several different mechanisms, including diminished need to monitor the partner's actions and benevolent attributions for negative partner behavior (Holmes & Rempel, 1989). Eventually, we hypothesize that a sustained intimate relationship with a trustworthy partner may even change core working models or beliefs regarding self and others (Holmes, 2002). In other words, high trust may lead to an increase in the security of the individual's adult attachment orientation.

The final pathway in the relationship enhancement model is between relationship satisfaction or stability and health. A large literature documents the negative effects of divorce and the positive effects of marital satisfaction and stability on physical and mental health (e.g., Berkman & Breslow, 1983; Burman & Margolin, 1992; Fenwick & Barressi, 1981; Gove, 1973; Kiecolt-Glaser & Newton, 2001; Sherbourne & Hays, 1990; Verbrugge, 1979; Wickrama, Lorenz, Conger, & Elder, 1997). Thus, social support promotes physical and mental health through its ability to prevent relationship deterioration and dissolution.

In the following sections, we consider each component of the model in greater depth. Evidence that supports the role of attributions in perceived partner support is discussed first, followed by the influence of individual difference variables (attachment orientation and neuroticism) on various processes in the model. The relationship between social support and trust is discussed next, followed by a summary of evidence that documents the salutary effects of trust on relationship quality and stability. Finally, research that links marital quality and stability to mental and physical health is briefly summarized.

The Role of Attributions

In this section, we describe the role of attributions for social support behaviors in the development of beliefs that the partner is a reliable source of social support and can be trusted to provide care when needed. Later in the chapter, we describe a reciprocal feedback relationship between trust and attributions. A large literature documents the link between attributions for partner behavior and marital satisfaction and stability (e.g., Bradbury & Fincham, 1992; Fincham & Bradbury, 1987; Fincham, Bradbury, Aria, Byrne, & Karney, 1997; Karney & Bradbury, 2000). Thus, it is very important to understand antecedents of positive and negative attributions for partner behavior.

ATTRIBUTIONS AND PERCEIVED SOCIAL SUPPORT. According to our model, whether an act intended to be supportive is perceived as supportive depends on the attributions that the recipient makes for why support was offered. Attributions may be to factors internal to the partner (e.g., a loving personality) or external to the partner (e.g., pressure from other people). Attributions may be made to factors that are controllable by the partner (e.g., effort) or uncontrollable by the partner (e.g., lack of ability). Finally, attributions may be made to factors that are stable or unstable. Stable factors are those that are likely to endure over time (e.g., strongly held attitudes), whereas unstable factors are those that are not likely to endure over time (e.g., a bad mood). According to attribution theory, if people are consistent in their tendency to offer social support in times of stress, then over time the support they provide will be attributed to internal, controllable, and stable characteristics (Kelley, 1973). Supportive acts that are attributed to stable, internal characteristics of the partner, such as kindness or commitment, contribute to perceived social support (Fincham & Bradbury, 1990). By contrast, supportive acts that are attributed to external causes, like social pressure, or to unstable causes, like a transitory good mood, do not contribute to the perception that the partner is a reliable source of social support.

We have conducted a series of laboratory studies examining the impact of attributions for support behaviors on perceived social support (Hessling, 2001). Using both correlational and experimental methods, we have found that the attributions that people make for the support behaviors they receive from others play a critical role in the extent to which they perceive the other's actions as supportive. Only support behaviors that are attributed to internal, controllable, and stable characteristics of the support provider are perceived as supportive (Hessling). Additional support for a link between attributions and perceived partner support comes from a study by Gallo and Smith (2001). They found that attributions for both positive and negative spouse behavior were strong predictors of perceived social support from the spouse. Significant correlations between attributions and perceived support were found in two additional studies (Brewin, MacCarthy, & Furnham, 1989; Mallinckrodt, 1992), although this association was not significant in a study by Slack and Vaux (1988). We argue, therefore, that attributions for partner support behaviors are important determinants of whether these behaviors are experienced as supportive. People's overall perceptions of partner supportiveness will grow to the extent that they believe that support is motivated by internal, stable, and controllable characteristics of the partner.

The Role of Individual Difference Variables

In an ideal world, when people consistently provide social support to their partner in times of stress, their partner will attribute these behaviors to internal and stable personality characteristics, such as generosity or caring. Furthermore, their partner will perceive them as a reliable source of support. Unfortunately, this is not always the case. In the relationship enhancement model of social support, we argue that individual difference variables influence attributions for supportive behaviors and perceptions of overall partner supportiveness. Two specific individual difference variables, adult attachment orientation and neuroticism, are hypothesized to influence support perceptions. Our focus on adult attachment orientation and neuroticism does not mean that other individual difference variables are irrelevant to the interpretation of supportive acts and perceived social support. However, to date, the largest and most consistent body of empirical evidence supports the influence of neuroticism and attachment orientation on processes and outcomes in intimate relationships (e.g., Karney & Bradbury, 1995). Furthermore, although we have portrayed attachment orientation and neuroticism as separate constructs, there is evidence that they are related (Carver, 1997; Shaver & Brennan, 1992) and may operate through at least some common mechanisms (Davila, Bradbury, & Fincham, 1998).

ATTACHMENT STYLE. Attachment theory states that early experiences with caregivers lead people to develop beliefs about the availability of others in times of need and the extent to which they are worthy of love (Bowlby, 1969). These beliefs translate into attachment orientations, which are manifested as attitudes, emotions, and behaviors in intimate relationships during adulthood (Hazan & Shaver, 1987). Those with a secure attachment orientation are comfortable with closeness and trust others to be available when needed. Two primary types of insecure attachment orientations have been identified, anxious ambivalent and avoidant. Those with an anxious–ambivalent attachment orientation crave closeness, but find it difficult to trust that others truly care for them. Those with an avoidant attachment orientation fear or mistrust closeness and strive to keep themselves safe by staying emotionally distant from others. The distinctive working models or belief systems associated with each attachment orientation influence how people evaluate the behavior of others (Collins, 1996; Gallo & Smith, 2001; Mikulincer & Florian, 1995; Whisman & Allan, 1996). A number of studies have documented a correlation between adult attachment orientation and perceived social support (Florian, Mikulincer, & Bucholtz, 1995; Hazan & Shaver, 1987; Kobak & Sceery, 1988; Ognibene & Collins, 1998). Studies have consistently found a positive association between security of attachment orientation and perceived social support.

Attributions for support are also influenced by adult attachment style and may be one mechanism through which attachment style influences perceptions of social support. Gallo and Smith (2001) found that for husbands, both anxious–ambivalent and avoidant attachment orientations predicted the tendency to make negative attributions for their wife's behavior. Furthermore, the authors found that negative attributions for the wife's behavior mediated the association between attachment orientation and perceived social support from the wife. It appears that the distinctive interpersonal schemas or belief systems that characterize anxious–ambivalent and avoidant attachment orientations influenced cognitions about the wife's behavior in a way that diminished men's ability to feel supported by their wives. Evidence for cognitive mediation of the link between attachment orientation and perceived social support has been found in other studies as well (Anders & Tucker, 2000; Fraley & Shaver, 1998).

NEUROTICISM. A number of studies have found a negative relation between neuroticism and perceived social support (e.g., Bolger & Eckenrode, 1991; Cutrona, Hessling, & Suhr, 1997; Halamandaris & Power, 1999; Lakey & Cassady, 1990; Russell, Booth, Reed, & Laughlin, 1997; Sarason, Levine, Basham, & Sarason, 1983). Our research group found that neuroticism predicted both overall perceived social support and attributions for specific support behaviors (Russell et al., 2000; Hessling, 2001). More specifically, neuroticism appeared to influence attributions for specific support interactions through the mediation of generalized cognitions regarding the availability of social support. Those who were high on neuroticism perceived low levels of social support from their social networks. In turn, perceptions of low availability of social support predicted negative attributions for actual support received during laboratory interactions. These results were replicated among dating couples and a sample of close-friend dyads (Russell et al., 2000). It appears that the more general tendency to interpret the world negatively is manifested in the expectation that network support will not be forthcoming in times of need. Negative beliefs about support from others predicted the tendency to attribute supportive acts to external factors rather than to genuine caring.

What are the implications of these findings for support in intimate relationships? Both adult attachment style and neuroticism appear to influence core beliefs about the availability of and motives behind social support from others. Thus, even a very supportive spouse may have difficulty convincing a partner with an insecure attachment style and/or high neuroticism that he or she can be relied on in times of duress. As we describe later in the chapter, therapeutic interventions for individuals who perceive low levels of support from their spouse may have to address both actual behavior *and* core beliefs about the availability of care from others.

The Role of Trust

The key prediction of the relationship enhancement model is that social support builds trust in intimate relationships. According to Holmes (2002), trust is the most important component of close relationships. A similar senti- ment was expressed by Berscheid (1994). Holmes and Berscheid both argue that beliefs about the partner's availability in times of need are central to eval- uations of overall relationship quality. In this section, we first present evidence that marital social support predicts trust. Next, we summarize evidence concerning the relation between trust and attributions for partner behavior and describe a process in which trust facilitates marital quality through the mediation of benign attributions for negative partner behaviors. After that, we argue that trust in one's intimate partner can increase the security of adult attachment orientation. Finally, we present empirical evidence that links trust to marital quality and stability.

TRUST AND SOCIAL SUPPORT. The relationship enhancement model of social support posits that a sustained pattern of supportive behaviors from the spouse facilitates the development of trust and the pervasive expectation that the spouse places high value on one's welfare. According to the relationship enhancement model, demonstrations of the partner's support are most critical during times of stress. When people are vulnerable, they experience the greatest need for assistance and reassurance.

It is surprising that previous models of the development of trust in intimate relationships have not included social support. These models have focused on acts of accommodation (inhibiting the urge to retaliate for negative partner behavior and instead responding in a pro-social manner) and acts of self-sacrifice for the sake of the relationship (Holmes, 2002; Rusbult, Verette, Whitney, Slovik, & Lipkus, 1991; Wieselquist, Rusbult, Agnew, & Foster, 1999). Social support behaviors share critical features with acts of self-sacri- fice and accommodation. Acts of social support frequently involve the decision to place the partner's welfare before one's own. For example, taking on addi- tional household tasks to allow the partner to complete an important work assignment involves sacrificing more personally attractive activities. Acts of social support sometimes involve accommodation. When people are coping with stressful life events, they often behave in unpleasant ways (Conger et al., 1990). Ignoring hostile remarks by the stressed partner and continuing to provide consistent emotional support is an example of accommodation.

We believe that social support provides the most direct evidence that one's partner will provide care in times of need. Social support behaviors con- stitute a large proportion of acts that demonstrate self-sacrifice and a signif- icant proportion of acts that demonstrate willingness to accommodate. Yet not all social support behaviors are subsumed under the categories of self-sacrifice or accommodation. Words of wise counsel, reassurance of the other's competence, expressions of empathy, and promises to *be there* for another through difficult times may be provided without self-sacrifice and without the rancor that sets the stage for accommodation. In sum, we argue that social support should be added to existing models of the development of trust in intimate relationships.

We recently tested the relationship enhancement model of social support in a longitudinal study of married couples recruited from university family housing (Cutrona, Russell, & Krebs, 2002). In this section, we report findings regarding the association between social support and trust. Couples came into the laboratory and took turns playing the role of discloser and support provider during two 10-minute conversations, one about a personal problem disclosed by the wife and one about a personal problem disclosed by the husband. We videotaped the interactions and later coded the behavior of the support provider using the Social Support Behavior Code (SSBC; Cutrona & Suhr, 1992; Suhr, Cutrona, Krebs, & Jensen, 2004). The SSBC is a microanalytic coding system that yields frequency counts of 23 types of supportive behaviors and 4 types of negative behavior (e.g., criticism and sarcasm). The codes are reduced to five summary scores: emotional support, esteem support, information support, tangible support and negative behavior. Emotional support includes expressions of caring and solidarity (e.g., "We will get through this together"). Esteem support includes expressions of encouragement and belief in the other's competence and ability (e.g., "You have more experience than any of the other applicants. I know you'll make a good impression in your interview"). Information support includes advice and factual input about the problem under discussion (e.g., "The main thing is not to let them see that you're anxious"). Finally, tangible support includes offers of resources or assistance (e.g., "I will take care of the baby all weekend so you can work on your dissertation").

Couples also completed self-report measures of perceived social support from the spouse, trust in the spouse, and marital quality. Both short- and long-term follow-ups were conducted, at 1 year and 7 years after the initial assessment (when the support interactions were videotaped). All of the questionnaire measures were repeated at the follow-up assessments.

Turning first to the observational measures, we found that the number of emotional support behaviors provided during the interaction predicted change in trust over a 1-year period. Individuals who received a high level of emotional support from their partner during the laboratory support interaction experienced an increase in trust over the following year. None of the other observed support or negative behavior codes predicted changes in trust. Furthermore, none of the observed support or negative behavior codes predicted trust at the 7-year follow-up.

We next conducted analyses to determine the extent to which changes in *perceived* spousal social support predicted changes in trust. As predicted, change in perceived support from the spouse significantly predicted change in trust. Those who experienced an increase in perceived social support from their spouse also experienced an increase in trust. This pattern was found both over the 1-year and the 7-year time periods.

Thus, our results showed significant relationships between spousal social support and trust, using both observational and self-report measures of social support. It is notable that the only social support behavior code that predicted future increases in trust was emotional support (expressions of caring, empathy, and solidarity). Instrumental support (advice and tangible assistance) was not related to partner trust. Thus, it appears that emotionally targeted support plays a greater role in building cognitions of trustworthiness than assistance with specific tasks.

TRUST AND ATTRIBUTIONS. According to Holmes (2002), attributional processes are influenced by trust. When trust is high, negative partner behaviors are relegated to low levels of importance by attributing them to unstable, external causes, such as stress at work or temporary forgetfulness (Holmes & Rempel, 1989). Thus, negative partner behaviors do not elicit intense emotional reactions or conflict. This is because the negative behavior is viewed as an aberration, not part of a pervasive pattern. Positive partner behaviors, by contrast, are attributed to internal and stable causes, which further strengthens the belief that the partner's motives toward oneself are positive.

The link between trust and attributions for undesirable partner behavior is extremely important. An extensive body of research documents the importance of attributions for negative partner behavior to marital quality (e.g., Fincham & Bradbury, 1987; Fincham et al., 1997; Karney & Bradbury, 2000; Kayser, 1993). When negative behaviors are attributed to stable, controllable characteristics of the spouse, such as meanness or selfishness, conflicts escalate in frequency and intensity and relationship quality deteriorates. When negative behaviors are attributed to unstable, external, or uncontrollable causes, conflicts do not escalate to the same extent and relationship quality is preserved. In a daily diary study of married couples, emotional reactivity to marital arguments was greater among wives with low levels of marital trust than among those with high levels of trust (Almeida, McGonagle, Cate, Kessler, & Wethington, 2003). Presumably, women with high levels of marital trust did not become as upset because they attributed the partner's behaviors during the conflict to benign rather than blameworthy causes. Similar results were reported by Frazier and colleagues, who found that negative partner behaviors only increased emotional distress among those with low marital satisfaction (Frazier, Tix, & Barnett, 2003). Among those with high marital satisfaction, negative partner behaviors had little impact on distress. Presumably, those with high marital satisfaction were also high on trust and attributed their partner's behavior to unstable and or external factors, thus neutralizing their destructive impact.

The association between trust and benign attributions for negative behaviors by the partner was demonstrated in a series of studies by Holmes and Rempel. In laboratory studies, they found that level of trust influenced both private and public attributions for partner behavior (Holmes & Rempel, 1989; Rempel et al., 1985; Rempel, Ross, & Holmes, 2001). When trust was high, negative partner behaviors were explained in a benevolent manner (attributed to external, unstable causes). When trust was low, negative partner behaviors were explained as blameworthy (attributed to internal, stable causes).

We extended this line of inquiry in our study of married students to determine whether trust predicts attributions for partner behavior over time. As described earlier, we assessed perceived spousal support and trust at all three times. At the third interview, we added a measure of attributions for positive and negative partner behaviors. Participants were given three positive spouse behaviors (e.g., "Your partner compliments you") and three negative spouse behaviors (e.g., "Your partner criticizes something you do") and asked to rate their attributions for each behavior with respect to stability and locus of causality (whether the cause was internal vs. external to the partner). As reported previously, we found that an increase in perceived social support predicted an increase in trust over the year from the first to the second assessment. We predicted that, in turn, trust at the second assessment would predict benign attributions for partner behavior at the third assessment, which was 7 years after the initial assessment.

Results were consistent with the relationship enhancement model. Both Time 2 trust and change in trust from Time 2 to Time 3 predicted scores on the measure of attributions for partner behavior. Those who reported a high level of trust in their partner at Time 2 and those who reported increasing trust from Time 2 to Time 3 reported benign attributions for their partner's negative behavior at Time 3. Benign attributions were those that explained the partner's negative behavior as the result of unstable and/or external causes, such as pressures at work or a bad mood. Contrary to prediction, trust did not predict attributions for positive partner behavior.

To summarize, level of trust plays an important role in shaping how undesirable partner behaviors are interpreted. When trust is low, undesirable behaviors are attributed to enduring characteristics of the partner and negative interactions occur at high rates of frequency and intensity. By contrast, when trust is high undesirable behaviors are attributed to causes that are unstable or external to the partner. Negative interactions occur with less intensity and frequency. Positive behaviors are interpreted as evidence of love and commitment. Thus, a positive spiral is created that enhances marital quality and stability.

TRUST AND ATTACHMENT ORIENTATION. Holmes (2002) argues that the "felt security" that results from the belief that one's partner can be counted on and will be responsive to one's needs is a critical ingredient in well-being. Furthermore, the experience of a trustworthy partner may change core beliefs about self and others. According to attachment theory, experiences with early caregivers lead to "internal working models" or beliefs about the availability of others and the extent to which one is worthy of love (Bowlby, 1969). According to the theory, these beliefs may be modified in adulthood through experiences with an intimate partner. Thus, over time, experiences with a trustworthy partner may lead to an increasingly secure adult attachment orientation. Those with a secure attachment orientation believe that others will be available when needed and that they themselves are worthy of love. They are comfortable with closeness and derive comfort from the presence of their intimate partner (Hazan & Shaver, 1987). There is mounting evidence that a secure attachment orientation is associated with relationship quality and stability (e.g., Feeney, 1996; Kobak & Hazan, 1991). Trust may thus strengthen intimate relationships both directly and indirectly through its impact on attachment orientation.

TRUST AND MARITAL QUALITY. Empirical evidence supports the relation between trust and marital quality. Both in dating and marital relationships, trust was associated with increased relationship satisfaction, poorer perceived quality of alternatives (i.e., alternatives to the current partner), and increased willingness to invest in the relationship in a study by Wieselquist et al. (1999). Additional evidence for the salutary effects of trust on relationship quality comes from Kurdek (2002), who found that both initial level and change in trust over an 8-year period predicted change in marital quality and marital separation. Couples who reported high levels of trust for their partner as new-lyweds and those whose trust increased over time reported high levels of marital satisfaction 8 years later. Couples who reported low levels of trust as newlyweds were more likely to have separated within the first 4 years of marriage. Declines in trust over time predicted a greater likelihood of separa-tion by the 8-year follow-up. Similarly, trust was a strong predictor of marital adjustment in another study of newlyweds (Quinn & Odell, 1998), and mutual trust was identified as one of the characteristics most likely to characterize long-lasting and satisfying marriages in a study of Israeli couples who had been married for more than 25 years (Sharlin, 1996).

Relationship Stability, Quality, and Health

The social support construct derives importance from its association with mental and physical health. We claim that an important mechanism through which social support affects health is through its ability to enhance relation-ship quality and prevent relationship dissolution. Thus, it is important to present evidence that relationship quality and stability are empirically linked to mental and physical health.

A large literature supports a connection between marital status and health. Compared with those who are married or cohabiting, the unmarried tend to have higher age-adjusted mortality rates from all causes (e.g., Berkman & Breslow, 1983; Lund et al., 2002). Those who are not married tend to rate their physical health less positively than those who are married (Kiecolt-Glaser & Newton, 2001; Ren, 1997; Ross, Mirowsky, & Goldsteen, 1990; Wyke & Ford, 1992). Mental health measures also show poorer adjust-ment for unmarried than married persons (e.g., Gove, Hughes, & Style, 1983; Wyke & Ford). It should be noted, however, that greater mental and physical health differences are found between married and divorced or separated persons than between married and never-married persons (Ren, 1997; Wyke & Ford, 1992). Marital disruption appears to have more deleterious effects on well-being than never marrying (Aseltine & Kessler, 1993).

A sizable literature documents the association between marital quality and mental health (e.g., Barnett, Brennan, Raudenbush, & Marshall, 1994; Cleary & Mechanic, 1983; Coyne, Thompson, & Palmer, 2002; Dehle & Weiss,

1998; Kurdek, 1998; McLeod & Eckberg, 1993; Wyke & Ford, 1992). Much less research has examined marital quality as a predictor of physical health, but growing evidence suggests that such a link exists. In a nationally representative sample of married and cohabiting adults, Ren (1997) found that those who reported being unhappy in their relationship were 1.39 times more likely to report poor physical health than those who were happy in their relationship. A prospective study of married women showed that over a 14-year period, marital satisfaction was negatively correlated with amount of atherosclerosis that developed in major blood vessels (Gallo et al., 2003) and other cardiovascular health risk factors (Gallo, Troxel, Matthews, & Kuller, 2003).

Wyke and Ford (1992) attempted to uncover mediators of the relation between marital status and health. As noted above, the greatest health differences are found between married and divorced or separated individuals. In their study, over 50% of the physical health differences between married and separated or divorced women and 38% of the differences for men were explained by perceived social support. The magnitude of the effect for social support was somewhat weaker than the effect of financial strain but much stronger than health risk behaviors in the prediction of physical health. Thus, the quality of perceived support appeared to play a significant role in the physical health of married versus separated and divorced individuals.

The association over time between marital quality and physical health was examined in a study of rural couples (Wickrama et al., 1997). Marital quality and number of physical health conditions (weighted by severity) were assessed three times at yearly intervals. For both husbands and wives, the initial level of marital quality and changes in marital quality over time predicted initial health status and changes in physical health conditions. Those whose marital quality was highest at the first assessment had higher initial health and less decline in health over time. Those whose marital quality improved reported improved physical health, whereas those whose marital quality declined reported declining physical health. These associations retained significance after controlling for the influence of income, education, and work stress. The association between marital quality and health was largely mediated by psychological well-being and health risk behaviors. Those in high quality marriages were less distressed and engaged in fewer health risk behaviors (e.g., smoking and lack of exercise). In turn, lower distress and fewer health risk behaviors predicted better health.

Finally, Robles and Kiecolt-Glaser (2003) examined the physiological effects of marital discord. They outlined a series of studies showing that conflict in married couples can trigger a series of deleterious physiological processes including an increase in both heart rate and stress hormones and a weakening of the immune system. These bodily changes were especially apparent in couples whose interactions were marked by hostility or other undesirable communication patterns. Couples who expressed themselves more constructively during conflict showed markedly less severe physiological responses.

In sum, there appears to be empirical support linking intimate relationship stability and quality with health. The link is better established between relationship variables and mental health; however, data suggest that psychological distress may mediate the relationship between relationship variables and physical health (Wickrama et al., 1997) and that hostility during conflict may be especially deleterious to physical health (Robles & Kiecolt-Glaser, 2003).

Illustrations of Key Processes

Because the relationship enhancement model has been presented in largely abstract terms, we thought it would be useful to offer illustrations of how various processes in the model manifest themselves in the lives of different couples. A best-case scenario is presented first (Couple A). In this couple, the personalities of both partners promote benign attributions and facilitate trust. To demonstrate the applicability of the model to same-sex as well as opposite-sex couples, a lesbian couple is used to illustrate this scenario. A less optimal scenario is presented second (Couple B). One member of the couple brings to the relationship personal characteristics that impede the development of trust. The final scenario illustrates the breakdown of support processes in two people who bring significant personal liabilities to the relationship (Couple C).

COUPLE A. Both Gina and Renee were raised by sensitive caregivers and brought a secure attachment orientation and low neuroticism to their relationship. Early in their relationship, they encountered considerable stress as both families had some difficulty adjusting to the reality of their daughters' sexual orientation. However, Gina and Renee were consistently supportive to one another through this period of turmoil. As time went on, family relationships improved and Gina and Renee were accepted as life partners by siblings and parents. The experience of finding consistent support from each other when families behaved in a hurtful manner led Gina and Renee to attribute each other's supportive behaviors to stable, controllable, and internal traits, including genuine caring, kindness, and commitment. Over time, Gina and Renee encountered a range of educational and interpersonal stressors. Although not perfect, their relationship was characterized by mutual respect, assistance, and encouragement. Each perceived the other as her primary source of social support. Over the years, trust grew and love deepened. At one point, Gina experienced a year of unwanted unemployment. She found this highly stressful, and it was difficult to hide her distress and resentment over the loss of her job. Because Renee trusted that Gina's core motives toward her were positive, she attributed Gina's occasional sharp-edged comments and lack of attentiveness to an external, unstable cause: the stress imposed by her unemployment. Renee ignored most of Gina's negative outbursts and provided encouragement, affection, and whatever tangible assistance was needed, such as paying bills for which Gina had previously been responsible. Eventually, Gina found meaningful employment, and the emotional tone of the relationship improved dramatically. Gina and Renee enjoyed a deeply rewarding relationship that endured throughout their lifetime. Although there were difficult phases in their relationship, they never considered termination. They watched with sadness as many of their friends' relationships dissolved and friends struggled with depression and stress-related disorders.

COUPLE B. Ruth and Tom were married a year after they graduated from college. Ruth came from a difficult family background. Her mother was alcoholic and found it difficult to provide nurturance to her daughter. In adulthood, Ruth found it difficult to trust others and avoided intimacy in most relationships, signs of an avoidant attachment orientation. Tom was luckier and emerged from a happy childhood with an outgoing personality and a secure attachment orientation. Tom and Ruth both found jobs that they liked after graduation. Tom found Ruth's distant manner disturbing but tried to be patient with her. He was mystified by her tendency to isolate herself rather than seek his aid when she was upset. Ruth found Tom's efforts to be supportive but unsettling. She was uncomfortable revealing vulnerability and viewed his attempts at support as intrusive. She accused him of trying to control her by giving her unwanted advice. Tom was hurt by her accusations. Over time, he learned to provide support unobtrusively. He quietly carried Ruth's load of housework during her busiest times at work. When she appeared distressed, he allowed her a period of withdrawal before asking her to disclose the source of her distress. He was careful to communicate his faith in her ability to solve her own problems. Gradually, Tom's strategy of providing support that was not threatening to Ruth's sense of autonomy was successful. Ruth slowly came to attribute Tom's supportive behaviors to stable, positive attributes of his personality and feelings toward her. Trust gradually increased. Eventually, her core beliefs about the availability of others in times of need shifted somewhat, although she remained distant toward all but Tom and a few close friends. Tom and Ruth decided not to have children and continued to make good progress in their careers. They traveled frequently and developed joint interests. The marriage lasted and was a source of meaningful companionship to both.

COUPLE C. After dating through their last 2 years of high school, Eleanor and Aaron were married during their first year of college. Eleanor had become pregnant, which led them to marry sooner than they had intended. Both Eleanor and Aaron were emotionally labile, personally insecure, and possessive, traits consistent with an anxious–ambivalent attachment orientation. Aaron had an especially negative outlook on the world and tended to be anxious and pessimistic, all signs of neuroticism or negative affectivity. Eleanor's pregnancy was a crisis to both Eleanor and Aaron. Each blamed the other. In their anger, neither was able to provide support to the other. Neither family was able to help the couple financially, so Aaron and Eleanor both dropped out of college. Aaron worked full time at a retail outlet, and Eleanor stayed home with the baby. Financial problems were ever present. Although both wanted to make the marriage work, exhaustion, worry, and frustration colored their interactions, which were rarely supportive and frequently accusatory. Problems were blamed on the negligence or incompetence of the other. Perceived support and trust remained low. Conflicts increased in bitterness and frequency. After the baby's third birthday, they separated and divorced. Both experienced significant depressive symptoms and life remained difficult for both.

ANALYSIS. In the first example, Gina and Renee were favored with dispositions that facilitated giving and receiving support from the other. They were able to develop trust and tolerance for the other's failings. In the second example, by contrast, Ruth found it very difficult to trust her husband, because experiences in early childhood left her with an avoidant attachment orientation. The secure attachment orientation of her partner made it possible for Ruth to become less guarded, make positive attributions for Tom's support, and become more trusting and less avoidant over time. In the third example, Eleanor and Aaron found it very difficult to trust each other because of their anxious–ambivalent attachment orientation and neuroticism. When faced with chronic financial stress, they were unable to give or receive support. Trust did not develop and the relationship dissolved. Both faced stress-related emotional disorders that may also increase risk for physical problems.

Implications of the Model

Implications for Theory

The relationship enhancement model of social support highlights a neglected mechanism in the process through which supportive acts influence health. Stated in the most general terms, social support enhances the quality and stability of intimate relationships, which in turn, enhance health. Part of support's effect is through the prevention of emotionally costly separation and divorce. Part is through diminished intensity and frequency of conflict, which results from increased trust. Both divorce and ongoing conflictual relationships are highly stressful and have negative stress-mediated health consequences. In addition, we believe that some of the health benefits of social support derive from the creation of relationships in which basic needs for connection and security are met (Holmes, 2002; Weiss, 1974). Through its enhancement of trust, social support allows people to let down their guard and "just enjoy the relationship" (Holmes, p. 20). Although the physiology of positive emotions is not well understood, it seems likely that positive affect has health-promoting effects beyond the mere absence of negative emotion.

The relationship enhancement model adopts a longer time frame than the buffering model of social support regarding the effects of support behaviors on health. The process of building trust takes time. Thus, the effects of supportive behaviors on health are expected to be delayed. By contrast, the buffering model highlights more immediate results of protection from the deleterious effects of stressful life events. If, in fact, the most important contribution of social support is to diminish rates of relationship dissolution, then among married individuals, the effects of early supportive behaviors in a relationship should show up most strongly at times of highest risk for divorce.

Highlighting the importance of causal attributions for supportive acts may provide some insight into the puzzling lack of correspondence between rate of received social support and level of perceived social support (Dunkel-Schetter & Bennett, 1990; Wethington & Kessler, 1986). Some acts of social support provided by members of the social network may be construed as compelled by duty or guilt rather than by genuine caring. Because they are not attributed to positive and stable characteristics of the provider, they do not contribute to perceptions of the individual as a reliable source of support.

The relationship enhancement model of social support interfaces with and extends previous work on the role of attributions in marital interaction and satisfaction. Trust, core beliefs about the partner's positive motives toward oneself, is viewed as an important determinant of the attributions that are made for the partner's negative behaviors. When trust is low, each action by the partner is closely scrutinized for possible evidence of hurtful or selfish intent. Thus, the rate of attributions is high as well as the negative content of attributions made for partner behavior. When trust is high, vigilance is relaxed and fewer partner behaviors are even analyzed with respect to intent. The rate of attributions is lower and the attributions made for negative behaviors are more benign (Holmes & Rempel, 1989). Thus, it may be worthwhile to incorporate the trust construct into models of attributions and relationship quality

As noted above, previous models of the antecedents of trust in close relationships have overlooked the contributions of social support. These models have focused on acts of self-sacrifice and accommodation. Some social support behaviors may be construed as evidence of the partner's willingness to sacrifice self-interest for the sake of the relationship. Others provide evidence that partner transgressions can be overlooked. However, consistent demonstrations of caring and concern in times of stress and adversity demonstrate a commitment to the partner's well-being that are not necessarily characterized by self-sacrifice or accommodation. The easy and spontaneous flow of these demonstrations of support may be part of their impact on trust.

Finally, the relationship enhancement model may enrich understanding of mechanisms through which adult attachment orientations affect social behavior and evaluations of others. To date, attachment theories have focused on attachment orientation as a determinant of the ability to trust. One contribution of the relationship enhancement model is its focus on a specific manifestation of low trust: the tendency to make negative attributions for positive and negative partner behaviors (Gallo & Smith, 2001). If positive behaviors are not attributed to stable, internal characteristics of the partner, they will not contribute to perceived social support. This pattern is consistent with the association of anxious–ambivalent and avoidant attachment orientations with low perceived social support (e.g., Florian et al., 1995). If negative behaviors are attributed to stable, internal causes, they take on increased import and trigger retaliatory negative behavior. This pattern is consistent with the association between insecure attachment orientation and maladaptive conflict behavior (e.g., Simpson, Rholes, & Phillips, 1996). Further research on the relation between adult attachment style and attributional processes is needed.

Implications for Intervention

Cutrona (1996) has argued that timing is a critical component of effectively implementing social-support-focused interventions. Social support is probably most effective in preventive interventions, such as premarital counseling. Providing individuals with a wide repertoire of supportive responses, educating them about the value of nurturant support (listening, encouraging, and empathizing rather than giving advice), and helping them to understand their partner's support preferences can set new relationships on a positive course (Cutrona). Early in the relationship, supportive behaviors are more likely to be interpreted as evidence of stable, positive partner characteristics than later in the relationship, when lack of support skill may have led to failures of support provision and erosion of trust.

A second context in which preventive social support interventions can be effective is at the onset of a crisis, such as the diagnosis of a serious illness in one member of the couple (see chap. 9, this volume). Severe life events often lead to deterioration in the quality of social support communication (see chaps. 2 & 5, this volume; Conger et al., 1990). To prevent the erosion of perceived support and trust, preventive interventions that help people maintain a high level of support for one another during times of crisis are needed. An excellent example of this kind of preventive intervention is the Couples Coping Enhancement Training (see chap. 8, this volume).

Social support skills training is not irrelevant to the treatment of troubled marriages. However, it is unlikely that simply teaching social support skills will be effective when anger, hurt, and suspicion over the partner's goodwill are high. Support behaviors enacted in this context will be discounted by attributions to therapist instructions or other external unstable causes (Jacobson & Margolin, 1979). Some restoration of trust is important before couples can convincingly begin to provide support to one another (Cutrona, 1996).

Interventions to increase perceived support in close relationships cannot be focused exclusively on skill building. The tendency of those who have low levels of perceived support to discount the supportive acts of others (Ross et al., 1999; Russell et al., 2000) suggests that cognitions about social support must also be addressed in therapy. The inadequacy of increasing the supply of social support to stressed individuals without addressing cognitions that limit receptivity to support was supported in a literature review of interventions to strengthen natural support networks (Cutrona & Cole, 2000). Interventions that provided coaching to network members on how to increase the support they provided to a stressed individual but did not also provide assistance to the stress victim about how to interpret and react to support did not succeed (see chaps. 5 & 9, this volume). The interventions that were most likely to succeed simultaneously addressed the supply of support and the cognitions of the recipient (e.g., Brand, Lakey, & Berman, 1995).

Because stable dispositions, such as attachment orientation and neuroticism, influence key processes in the translation of social support into relationship quality and health, therapeutic interventions will vary in how successful they are, depending on the characteristics of the participants. Those with insecure attachment orientations and/or high neuroticism will find it more difficult to make positive attributions for their partner's behavior, to perceive their partner as a reliable source of social support, and to trust their partner. One reason that attribution-focused therapy programs have met with limited success may be the intractability of attributional tendencies that are rooted in deep-seated working models and negative affectivity and neuroticism.

Implications for Research

Three recommendations for how to assess social support in future studies emerge from the relationship enhancement model. The first is that measures of social support that do not delineate specific sources of support be used less frequently and only when the intent is to access very general schemas of support availability. The relationship enhancement model posits that an important ingredient in the link between social support and health is the development and preservation of intimate relationships. Further tests of this link require that received and perceived support from the intimate partner be assessed separately from support derived from other sources. The second recommendation is that greater use be made of observational methods for assessing social support in the transactions of intimate partners. To understand the nature of successful support communications, it is important to analyze actual transactions between partners. Marital therapy benefited from careful analysis of the conflict behaviors of distressed versus nondistressed couples. Interventions focused on decreasing the maladaptive behaviors seen among the distressed couples and increasing the constructive behaviors seen among nondistressed couples. Social support interventions should also be built on empirical observations of the communication content and style of couples who are successful versus unsuccessful in communicating support and building trust. Communication strategies that impede support can be discouraged and those that facilitate support can be reinforced. Finally, because it is not simply support behaviors that generate perceived support and trust but also cognitions about those behaviors, we recommend studies in which behaviors and cognitions about support behaviors are assessed as predictors of the perceived supportiveness of dyadic interactions. Although the relationship enhancement model emphasizes causal attributions, other dimensions of cognition, including social comparison, cognitive dissonance, and expectation processes should be investigated as well.

Remaining Challenges

The relationship enhancement model has never been tested in its entirety. Instead, it has been assessed in a somewhat piecemeal fashion, relying on studies from a wide range of sources. No single study to date has included all of the component variables assessed repeatedly over a sufficient period of time with a sufficiently large sample to provide convincing evidence for the model's viability. This is, of course, a key goal for future research.

Theoretical questions remain unanswered as well. First, it is not clear that social support behaviors and resultant trust affect all of the components necessary to preserve intimate relationships. Passion is component that may or may not be influenced by the mechanisms described in the relationship enhancement model. It is not difficult to imagine a relationship in which partners both trust and are bored with one another. It may be that persons with different love styles may benefit differentially from support-based trust. Those who value companionate love are probably best situated to benefit from the processes described in this chapter. Those whose ideal relationship is characterized by high passion and excitement may not benefit from the calm of security and trust. On a related topic, social support processes may increase trust, but they may not be sufficient to kindle or rekindle love, one of the most difficult qualities to influence therapeutically (Geiss & O'Leary, 1981; Kayser, 1993). The issue of social support's influence or lack of influence on passion and love merits further consideration.

A second question left unanswered by the relationship enhancement model is the relative importance of skill versus intent in social support provision. It is possible that an individual may deeply value his or her partner's well-being but may be clumsy or insensitive in the communication of social support. For example, there is evidence that some kinds of social support are more effective than others following specific types of stressors (Cohen & McKay, 1984; Cutrona & Russell, 1990; Lanza, Cameron, & Revenson, 1995). If ill-chosen types of support are given, will they strengthen perceptions of perceived partner support? There is some evidence that benign attributions are frequently made for social support "mistakes" (Lehman & Hemphill, 1990), but repeated experiences of frustration over the ineffectiveness of well-intentioned social support may undermine the effect of support experiences on well-being.

Finally, the relationship enhancement model may not have included all of the pathways among variables. For example, attachment style and neuroticism may influence every step of the process from social support to health. The relationship enhancement model includes direct links between these characteristics and attributions for partner behavior and perceived social support. However, evidence also supports correlations of attachment style and neuroticism with other variables, including trust and marital outcomes (e.g., Karney & Bradbury, 1995; Kobak & Hazan, 1991). The extent to which such links are direct or mediated by other variables remains to be investigated further.

The theme of this volume is couples coping with stress. We have provided a new perspective on the long-range implications of how well or poorly couples support each other during difficult times. We have articulated some of the cognitive and individual-differences variables that we believe are important to this process. According to our model, the support provided during times of adversity has long-range implications, both for the relationship and for the health of both partners.

References

Almeida, D. M., McGonagle, K. A., Cate, R. C., Kessler, R. C., & Wethington, E. (2003). Psychosocial moderators of emotional reactivity to marital arguments: Results from a daily diary study. *Marriage and Family Review, 34*, 89–113.

Anders, S. L., & Tucker, J. S. (2000). Adult attachment style, interpersonal communication competence, and social support. *Personal Relationships, 7*, 379–389.

Aseltine, R. H., & Kessler, R. C. (1993). Marital disruption and depression in a community sample. *Journal of Health and Social Behavior, 34*, 237–251.

Barnett, R. C., Brennan, R. T., Raudenbush, S. W., & Marshall, N. L. (1994). Gender and the relationship between marital-role quality and psychological distress. *Psychology of Women Quarterly, 18*, 105–127.

Berkman, L. F., & Breslow, L. (1983). *Health and ways of living: The Alameda County Study.* New York: Oxford University Press.

Berscheid, E. (1994). Interpersonal relationships. *Annual Review of Psychology, 45,* 79–129.

Bolger, N., & Eckenrode, J. (1991). Social relationships, personality, and anxiety during a major stressful event. *Journal of Personality and Social Psychology, 61,* 440–449.

Bowlby, J. (1969). *Attachment and loss: Vol 1. Attachment.* New York: Basic Books.

Bradbury, T. N., & Fincham, F. D. (1992). Attributions and behavior in marital interaction. *Journal of Personality and Social Psychology, 63,* 613–628.

Brand, E. F., Lakey, B., & Berman, S. (1995). A preventive psychoeducational approach to increase social support. *American Journal of Community Psychology, 23,* 117–135.

Brewin, C. R., MacCarthy, B., & Furnham, A. (1989). Social support in the role of adversity: The role of cognitive appraisal. *Journal of Research in Personality, 23,* 354–372.

Burman, B., & Margolin, G. (1992). Analysis of the association between marital relationships and health problems: An interactional perspective. *Psychological Bulletin,* 112, 39–63.

Carver, C. S. (1997). Adult attachment and personality: Converging evidence and a new measure. *Personality and Social Psychology Bulletin, 23,* 865–883.

Cassel, J. B. (1976). The contribution of the social environment to host resistance. *American Journal of Epidemiology, 107,* 107–123.

Cleary, P. D., & Mechanic, D. (1983). Sex differences in psychological distress among married people. *Journal of Health and Social Behavior, 24,* 111–121.

Cobb, S. (1976). Social support as a moderator of life stress. *Psychosomatic Medicine, 38,* 300–314.

Cohen, S., & McKay, G. (1984). Social support, stress, and the buffering hypothesis: A theoretical analysis. In A. Baum, J. E. Singer, & S. E. Taylor (Eds.), *Handbook of psychology and health* (pp. 253–267). Hillsdale, NJ: Erlbaum.

Cohen, S., & Wills, T. (1985). Stress, social support, and the buffering hypothesis. *Psychological Bulletin, 98,* 310–357.

Collins, N. L. (1996). Working models of attachment: Implications for explanation, emotion, and behavior. *Journal of Personality and Social Psychology, 71,* 810–832.

Conger, R. D., Elder, G. H., Lorenz, F. O., Conger, K. J., Simons, R. L., Whitbeck, L. B., Huck, S., & Melby, J. N. (1990). Linking economic hardship to marital quality and instability. *Journal of Marriage and the Family, 52,* 643–656.

Coyne, J. C., Thompson, R., & Palmer, S. C. (2002). Marital quality, coping with conflict, marital complaints, and affection in couples with a depressed wife. *Journal of Family Psychology, 16,* 26–37.

Cutrona, C. E. (1996). *Social support in couples: Marriage as a resource in times of stress.* Thousand Oaks, CA: Sage.

Cutrona, C. E., & Cole, V. (2000). Optimizing support in the natural network. In L. G. Underwood, S. Cohen, & B. H. Gottlieb (Eds.), *Social support measurement and interventions: A guide for health and social scientists* (pp. 278–308). New York: Oxford University Press.

Cutrona, C. E., Hessling, R. M., & Suhr, J. A. (1997). The influence of husband and wife personality on marital social support interactions. *Personal Relationships, 4,* 379–393.

Cutrona, C. E., & Russell, D. W. (1990). Type of social support and specific stress: Toward a theory of optimal matching. In I. G. Sarason, B. R. Sarason, & G. Pierce (Eds.), *Social support: An interactional view* (pp. 319–366). New York: Wiley.

Cutrona, C. E., Russell, D. W., & Krebs, K. (2002, October). *Dimensions of behavior predicting marital outcomes.* Paper presented at the International Meeting on the Developmental Course of Couples Coping with Stress, Boston College, Boston, MA.

Cutrona, C. E., & Suhr, J. A. (1992). Controllability of stressful events and satisfaction with spouse support behaviors. *Communication Research, 19,* 154–176.

Davila, J., Bradbury, T. N., & Fincham, F. D. (1998). Negative affectivity as a mediator of the association between adult attachment and marital satisfaction. *Personal Relationships, 5,* 467–484.

Dehle, C., & Weiss, R. L. (1998). Sex differences in prospective associations between marital quality and depressed mood. *Journal of Marriage and the Family, 60,* 1002–1011.

Dunkel-Schetter, C., & Bennett, T. L. (1990). Differentiating the cognitive and behavioral aspects of social support. In B. R. Sarason, I. G. Sarason, & G. R. Pierce (Eds.), *Social support: An interactional view* (pp. 267–296). New York: Wiley.

Feeney, J. A. (1996). Attachment, caregiving, and marital satisfaction. *Personal Relationships, 3,* 401–416.

Fenwick, R., & Barresi, C. M. (1981). Health consequences of marital-status change among the elderly: A comparison of cross-sectional and longitudinal analyses. *Journal of Health and Social Behavior, 22,* 106–116.

Fincham, F. D., & Bradbury, T. N. (1987). The impact of attributions in marriage: A longitudinal analysis. *Journal of Personality and Social Psychology, 53*, 510–517.

Fincham, F. D., & Bradbury, T. N. (1990). Social support in marriage: The role of social cognition. *Journal of Social and Clinical Psychology, 9*, 31–42.

Fincham, F. D., Bradbury, T. N., Aria, I., Byrne, C. A., & Karney, B. R. (1997). Marital violence, marital distress, and attributions. *Journal of Family Psychology, 11*, 367–372.

Florian, V., Mikulincer, M., & Bucholtz, I. (1995). Effects of adult attachment style on the perception and search for social support. *Journal of Psychology, 129*, 665–676.

Fraley, R. C., & Shaver, P. R. (1998). Airport separations: A naturalistic study of adult attachment dynamics in separating couples. *Journal of Personality and Social Psychology, 75*, 1198–1212.

Frazier, P. A., Tix, A. P., & Barnett, C. L. (2003). The relational context of social support: Relationship satisfaction moderates the relations between enacted support and distress. *Personality and Social Psychology Bulletin, 29*, 1133–1146.

Gallo, L. C., & Smith, T. W. (2001). Attachment style in marriage: Adjustment and responses to interaction. *Journal of Social and Personal Relationships, 18*, 263–289.

Gallo, L. C., Troxel, W. M., Kuller, L. H., Sutton-Tyrrell, K., Edmundowicz, D., & Matthews, K. A. (2003). Marital status, marital quality, and atherosclerotic burden in postmenopausal women. *Psychosomatic Medicine, 65*, 952–962.

Gallo, L. C., Troxel, W. M., Matthews, K. A., & Kuller, L. H. (2003). Marital status and quality in middle-aged women: Associations with levels and trajectories of cardiovascular risk factors. *Health Psychology, 22*, 453–463.

Geiss, S. K., & O'Leary, D. (1981). Therapist ratings of frequency and severity of marital problems: Implications for research. *Journal of Marital and Family Therapy, 7*, 515–520.

Gove, W. R. (1973). Sex, marital status, and mortality. *American Journal of Sociology, 79*, 45–67.

Gove, W. R., Hughes, M., & Style, C. B. (1983). Does marriage have a positive effect on the psychological well-being of the individual? *Journal of Health and Social Behavior, 24*, 122–131.

Halamandaris, K. F., & Power, K. G. (1999). Individual differences, social support and coping with the examination stress: A study of the psychosocial and academic adjustment of first year home students. *Personality and Individual Differences, 26*, 665–685.

Hazan, C., & Shaver, P. R. (1987). Romantic love conceptualized as an attachment process. *Journal of Social and Personality Psychology, 52*, 511–524.

Hessling, R. M. (2001). An experimental investigation of the role of personality and attributions in influencing the evaluation of social support. *Dissertation Abstracts International, 61*(7), 3901B.

Holmes, J. G. (2002). Interpersonal expectations as the building blocks of social cognition: An interdependence theory perspective. *Personal Relationships, 9*, 1–26.

Holmes, J. G., & Rempel, J. K. (1989). Trust in close relationships. In C. Hendrick (Ed.), *Close relationships* (pp. 187–220). Newbury Park, CA: Sage.

Jacobson, N. S., & Margolin, G. (1979). *Marital therapy: Strategies based on social learning and behavior exchange principles*. New York: Brunner/Mazel.

Karney, B. R., & Bradbury, T. N. (1995). The longitudinal course of marital quality and stability: A review of theory, method, and research. *Psychological Bulletin, 118*, 3–34.

Karney, B. R., & Bradbury, T. N. (2000). Attributions in marriage: State of trait? A growth curve analysis. *Journal of Personality and Social Psychology, 78*, 295–309.

Kayser, K. (1993). *When love dies: The process of marital disaffection*. New York: Guilford Press.

Kelley, H. H. (1973). The processes of causal attribution. *American Psychologist, 34*, 107–128.

Kiecolt-Glaser, J. K., & Newton, T. L. (2001). Marriage and health: His and hers. *Psychological Bulletin, 127*, 472–503.

Kobak, R. R., & Hazan, C. (1991). Attachment in marriage: Effects of security and accuracy of working models. *Journal of Personality and Social Psychology, 60*, 861–869.

Kobak, R. R., & Sceery, A. (1988). Attachment in late adolescence: Working models, affect regulation, and representations of self and others. *Child Development, 59*, 134–146.

Kurdek, L. A. (1998). The nature and predictors of the trajectory of change in marital quality over the first four years of marriage for first-married husbands and wives. *Journal of Family Psychology, 12*, 494–510.

Kurdek, L. A. (2002). Predicting the timing of separation and marital satisfaction: An eight-year prospective longitudinal study. *Journal of Marriage and the Family, 64*, 163–170.

Lakey, B., & Cassady, P. B. (1990). Cognitive processes in perceived social support. *Journal of Personality and Social Psychology, 59*, 337–343.

Lanza, A. F., Cameron, A. E., & Revenson, T. A. (1995). Helpful and unhelpful support among individuals with rheumatic diseases. *Psychology & Health, 10,* 449–462.

Lehman, D. R., & Hamphill, K. J. (1990). Recipients' perceptions of support attempts and attributions for support attempts that fail. *Journal of Social and Personal Relationships, 7,* 563–574.

Lund, R., Due, P., Modvig, J., Holstein, B. E., Damsgaard, M. T., & Anderson, P. K. (2002). *Social Science and Medicine, 55,* 673–679.

Mallinckrodt, B. (1992). Childhood emotional bonds with parents, development of adult social competencies, and availability of social support. *Journal of Counseling Psychology, 39,* 453–461.

McLeod, J. D., & Eckberg, D. A. (1993). Concordance for depressive disorders and marital quality. *Journal of Marriage and the Family, 55,* 733–746.

Mikulincer, M., & Florian, V. (1995). Appraisal of and coping with a real-life stressful situation: The contribution of attachment style. *Personality and Social Psychology Bulletin, 21,* 406–414.

Ognibene, T. C., & Collins, N. L. (1998). Adult attachment styles, perceived social support, and coping strategies. *Journal of Social and Personal Relationships, 15,* 323–345.

Quinn, W. H., & Odell, M. (1998). Predictors of marital adjustment during the first two years. *Marriage and Family Review, 27,* 113–130.

Rempel, J. K., Holmes, J. G., & Zanna, M. P. (1985). Trust in close relationships. *Journal of Personality and Social Psychology, 49,* 95–112.

Rempel, J. K., Ross, M., & Holmes, J. G. (2001). Trust and communication attributions in close relationships. *Journal of Personality and Social Psychology, 81,* 57–64.

Ren, X. S. (1997). Marital status and quality of relationships: The impact on health perception. *Social Science and Medicine, 44,* 241–249.

Robles, T. F., & Kiecolt-Glaser, J. K. (2003). The physiology of marriage: Pathways to health. *Physiology & Behavior, 79,* 409–416.

Ross, C. E., Mirowsky, J., & Goldsteen, K. (1990). The impact of the family on health: The decade in review. *Journal of Marriage and the Family, 52,* 1059–1078.

Rusbult, C. E., Verette, J., Whitney, G. A., Slovik, L. F., & Lipkus, I. (1991). Accommodation processes in close relationships: Theory and preliminary empirical evidence. *Journal of Personality and Social Psychology, 60,* 53–78.

Russell, D. W., Booth, B., Reed, D., & Laughlin, P. R. (1997). Personality, social networks, and perceived social support among alcoholics: A structural equation analysis. *Journal of Personality, 65,* 649–692.

Russell, D. W., Hessling, R. M., & Cutrona, C. E. (2000, June). *Causal attributions and the perception of social support.* Paper presented at the Second Joint Conference of the International Society for Social and Personal Relationships and the International Network on Personal Relationships, University of Queensland, Brisbane, Australia.

Sarason, I. G., Levine, H. M., Basham, R. B., & Sarason, B. R. (1983). Assessing social support: The Social Support Questionnaire. *Journal of Personality and Social Psychology, 44,* 127–139.

Sharlin, S. A. (1996). Long-term successful marriages in Israel. *Contemporary Family Therapy, 18,* 225–242.

Shaver, P. R., & Brennan, K. A. (1992). Attachment styles and the "Big Five" personality traits: Their connections with each other and with romantic relationship outcomes. *Personality and Social Psychology Bulletin, 18,* 536–545.

Sherbourne, C. D., & Hays, R. D. (1990). Marital status, social support, and health transitions in chronic disease patient. *Journal of Health and Social Behavior, 31,* 328–343.

Simpson, J. A., Rholes, W. S., & Phillips, D. (1996). Conflict in close relationships: An attachment perspective. *Journal of Personality and Social Psychology, 71,* 899–914.

Slack, D., & Vaux, A. (1988). Undesirable life events and depression: The role of event appraisals and social support. *Journal of Social and Clinical Psychology, 7,* 290–296.

Suhr, J. A., Cutrona, C. E., Krebs, K., & Jensen, S. L. (2004). The Social Support Behavior Code. In P. K. Kerig & D. Baucom (Eds.), *Couple observational coding systems* (pp. 307–318). Mahwaw, NJ: Erlbaum.

Verbrugge, L. (1979). Marital status and health. *Journal of Marriage and the Family, 41,* 267–285.

Weiss, R. L. (1974). The provisions of social relations. In Z. Rubin (Ed.), *Doing unto others* (pp. 17–26). Engelwood Cliffs, NJ: Prentice Hall.

Wethington, E., & Kessler, R. C. (1986). Perceived support, received support, and adjustment to stressful life events. *Journal of Health and Social Behavior, 27,* 78–89.

Whisman, M. A., & Allan, L. E. (1996). Attachment and social cognition theories of romantic relationships: Convergent or complementary perspectives? *Journal of Social and Personal Relationships, 13,* 263–278.

Wickrama, K. A. S., Lorenz, F. O., Conger, R. D., & Elder, G. H. (1997). Marital quality and physical illness: A latent growth curve analysis. *Journal of Marriage and the Family, 59,* 143–155.

Wieselquist, J., Rusbult, C. E., Agnew, C. R., & Foster, C. A. (1999). Commitment, pro-relationship behavior, and trust in close relationships. *Journal of Personality and Social Psychology, 77,* 942–966.

Wyke, S., & Ford, G. (1992). Competing explanations for associations between marital status and health. *Social Science and Medicine, 34,* 523–532.

5

How Partners Talk in Times of Stress: A Process Analysis Approach

Nancy Pistrang and Chris Barker

> I kind of feel sometimes a bit stuck as to what is a good thing or not a good thing to do . . . We're kind of just stumbling along between the two of us, trying to solve things as we go along in whichever way we think is going to work for us . . . (Man whose partner was depressed)

> [It's like] walking on eggshells . . . I didn't know what to say to him, to make him feel better. But I was also afraid of saying anything at all because any little thing could have made him feel worse . . . It was very, very emotional and very upsetting for me to see him and to be trying to use the right words and . . . do the right things. It was very hard indeed. (Woman whose partner had been depressed)

This is how two people described their efforts to provide support when their partner was suffering from depression (Harris, Pistrang, & Barker, 2004). Like other couples interviewed in our study of partner support in depression, they expressed bewilderment, frustration, and sometimes, despair about the best way to help; there was a sense of having to proceed carefully and learn by trial and error.

When couples face difficult circumstances in their lives, how does one member of the couple attempt to help the other? How can we make sense of such helping interactions? And why study couples' helping interactions in the first place?

We aim in this chapter to provide some answers to these questions. In particular, we suggest a conceptual framework for studying couples' helping interactions and a methodological approach that allows an in-depth, idiographic examination of such interactions. We draw on data from our own studies of couples facing various life stresses, including breast cancer, heart disease, the transition to parenthood, and depression. The first section of the chapter presents the rationale for studying partners' helping interactions. The second and third sections outline our conceptual and methodological approaches, which are then illustrated by two extended case examples. Finally, we briefly consider how research on couples' helping interactions might be translated into interventions to maximize the support that partners can provide for each other.

Throughout this chapter we use the terms *partner* and *couple* to refer to people in intimate relationships, whether married or not. Although our own research has focused on helping interactions in heterosexual relationships, the approach we describe can be applied to same-sex couples as well as to other close relationships such as friendships.

Why Study Partner Support?

It is now almost a truism that support from others helps people adjust to life stresses. For those people in close relationships, support from the partner may be particularly important. Indeed, sociologists noted the *therapeutic* role of marital partners several decades ago (e.g., Blood & Wolfe, 1960; Nye, 1976). General population surveys of informal helping have shown that the partner is one of the most frequently used sources of help during times of stress (Barker, Pistrang, Shapiro, & Shaw, 1990; Veroff, Kulka, & Douvan, 1981).

Although only a small proportion of the social support literature has focused specifically on the partner, a number of studies have found that support from the partner is associated with psychological adjustment to various medical conditions (see reviews by Cutrona, 1996; Manne, 1998; chap. 6, this volume). Furthermore, at times of stress the partner's role may be pivotal: There is some evidence to suggest that support from other relationships may not compensate for the lack of a confiding relationship with the partner (Brown & Harris, 1978; Coyne & DeLongis, 1986; Pistrang & Barker, 1995).

Yet, even though the partner seems to be of central importance, we know that it is not always easy for partners to support each other. A number of authors have pointed to some particular difficulties that may arise when people are attempting to provide support within the context of a close relationship. As Coyne and colleagues have argued forcefully, support is not simply something that is given by one partner and received by the other: It occurs in the context of an ongoing, interdependent, relationship in which each partner has his or her own needs, goals, and emotions. Thus "dilemmas of helping" may arise from the dual tasks of trying to provide support for one's partner while at the same time trying to manage one's own needs (Coyne & DeLongis, 1986; Coyne, Ellard, & Smith, 1990). For example, a husband's efforts to reassure his wife that her breast cancer will not recur may be motivated by his need to reduce his own feelings of distress about her illness (Pistrang, Barker, & Rutter, 1997). On a similar note, Cutrona and Suhr (1994) have suggested that social support in couples be viewed in the context of the couple's efforts to strike a balance between interdependence and personal autonomy: How a support attempt is perceived may be influenced by the individual's needs for both closeness and autonomy.

Clearly, efforts to provide support do not always succeed. "Failed" support attempts by partners as well as other helpers are well documented (e.g., Dakof & Taylor, 1990; Lehman, Ellard, & Wortman, 1986). One aim of social support research has been to identify successful and unsuccessful support behaviors. However, despite a vast literature on social support, there is little empirical data to suggest that certain types of support behaviors are consistently helpful, while others are not. As many researchers have concluded, the impact of any support behavior is highly dependent on the context: The nature of the stressor, the particular needs of the recipient, and who the support provider is have all been shown to influence whether a behavior is perceived as supportive or not (e.g., Cutrona, 1996; Dakof & Taylor, 1990; Lanza, Cameron, & Revenson, 1995).

From a cognitive perspective, several researchers have also pointed to the importance of taking into account the recipient's appraisals of, or attributions for, the support provider's behavior, particularly in the context of close relationships. For example, Fincham and Bradbury (1990) suggest that explanations for spouse behavior (e.g., whether it is viewed as voluntary and selflessly motivated) may play a central role in determining whether the behavior is perceived as supportive. To ignore such contextual and cognitive variables risks oversimplifying the nature of support processes.

Despite this recognition of the complexity of social support, we still know relatively little about the processes of support in the context of close relationships. How do spouses interact when one partner is in need of support, and how are these interactions perceived? There are at least two reasons for our limited knowledge. First, with only a few exceptions, the vast bulk of the social support literature has relied on retrospective, self-report methods despite repeated calls over the last decade or so for a more interactional approach to the study of social support (Burleson, Albrecht, & Sarason, 1994; Sarason, Sarason, & Pierce, 1990). Although self-report instruments certainly have value, they are limited in what they can tell us about how partners actually communicate with each other. Second, research on couples' communication, which has a long tradition of using observational methods to investigate how couples interact, has focused almost exclusively on conflictual interactions (Bradbury, Fincham, & Beach, 2000). It is only recently that couples researchers have begun to examine supportive interactions (e.g., Pasch & Bradbury, 1998). By and large, these two literatures, social support and couples' communication, have remained largely separate, with little cross-fertilization.

The paucity of research on couples' supportive interactions has limited not only our understanding of effective (and ineffective) support processes but also the development of empirically based interventions for those couples who struggle to support each other during times of stress. A prerequisite for designing interventions is knowledge of what couples actually do when they attempt to help one another and how they construe such attempts. Given the centrality of the partner as a provider of support, surprisingly few social support interventions seem to have been targeted specifically at couples (e.g., Hogan, Linden, & Najarian, 2002; Milne, 1999; chap. 9, this volume).

We propose an alternative conceptual and methodological approach to studying how couples interact when facing life stresses. Our hope is that a different way of thinking about support may have the potential to stimulate both further research and the development of effective clinical interventions.

A Conceptual Framework for Studying Couples' Interactions

Although the social support field has moved toward taking a more interactional view of the phenomena under investigation, it has remained circumscribed by its original roots and terminology in the concept of *support*, a metaphor whose literal meaning denotes the activity of holding up, sustaining, or preventing collapse. Perhaps the deficiencies of this metaphor underlie some of the problems and limitations of the field.

We propose that a more fruitful approach might be to invoke the conceptual framework of *psychological helping* for studying support processes in general, and those within couples' relationships specifically (Barker & Pistrang, 2002). Broadly speaking, there is a continuum of psychological helping interactions, ranging from informal to formal (Cowen, 1982; Christensen & Jacobson, 1994). At one end of the continuum are the pure *informal helping* interactions, those that spontaneously arise in natural settings between people of roughly the same social status who have no or little background or training in psychological helping. Social support processes, including those occurring within couples' relationships, clearly come under this heading. At the other end of the continuum are the *formal helping* interactions, such as those that occur in psychotherapy, counseling, and guidance with high-status, trained helpers at prearranged times in official settings. Paraprofessional helping, peer support, mutual help groups, and mentoring programs (e.g., high school teachers or professors helping their students with nonacademic matters) occupy intermediate points of the continuum. The bulk of research examining psychological helping has concentrated on the formal helping end of the continuum: Many volumes and entire journals are devoted to the analysis of psychotherapy and counseling, whereas a comparatively miniscule literature exists on psychological helping in everyday relationships, particularly within couples.

One advantage of situating social support within the spectrum of psychological helping interactions is that it allows us to look for commonalties across the seemingly disparate manifestations of the phenomenon. It opens up the possibility for a mutually enriching cross-fertilization between the formal and informal helping literatures (Barker & Pistrang, 2002). In particular, scholars in the area of therapy and counseling research have built up a large corpus of literature on the ways of tackling problems that may well be of value to social support researchers.

Second, the helping metaphor, in contrast to the support metaphor, opens up the idea that interactions with others may lead to a process of change for the individual. Like the outcome of a successful psychotherapeutic interaction, informal helping may also permanently change, in a beneficial way, the person's outlook on life or their habitual way of coping with problems.

Process Research

One of the potential ways in which social support researchers could draw from the approaches used to study formal helping (i.e., psychotherapy and counseling) is to adapt some of the existing process research concepts. Process research focuses on the nature of the interactions between the helper and helpee (in contrast to outcome research, which examines the impact of these interactions). It is from the psychotherapy process research tradition that the work described in the current chapter derives.

A fundamental piece of terminology is the intention–response–impact sequence. Each verbal response that a helper makes (e.g., "Have you tried talking to your boss directly?") is said to have an intention (e.g., finding out information or trying to change behavior), and each helper response is said to have a psychological impact on the helpee (e.g., feeling criticized or seeing a new way to deal with a problem). These concepts are not unique to therapy research and provide a way of making distinctions that can untangle some of the complexities of helping processes. It is useful when studying such processes to ask three questions: (a) What is the helper trying to do (intention)? (b) What does the helper actually say or do (response)? and (c) What is the effect of the response on the helpee (impact)? The commonly used social support categories tend to blur these distinctions. For example, is *esteem support* a kind of support aimed at raising the person's self-esteem (intention), a kind of support containing reference to self-esteem (response), or a kind of support resulting in increased self-esteem (impact)? A clearer specification of what is being referred to makes it easier to understand helping processes, particularly as intention does not always correspond to impact.

Other useful ideas drawn from process research are the conceptualization of generic variables that describe the important aspects of helping interactions. We elaborate on this in the following section.

Components of Helping

On the face of it, there is a bewildering number of different orientations to psychological therapies and counseling: psychoanalysis, cognitive–behavioral therapy, Gestalt therapy, and client-centered therapy being some of the most popular. However, many scholars have postulated that underneath this apparent diversity lie some common, pan-theoretical principles that underpin all therapeutic interactions. That is, generic processes may operate across all of the many different orientations. This is the so-called *common factors* explanation: that similar factors may explain the effectiveness of a number of different approaches to psychological helping (Hubble, Duncan, & Miller, 1999; Stiles, Shapiro, & Elliott, 1986).

One goal of the early process researchers, particularly that of the pioneering work of Carl Rogers and his group at the University of Chicago in the 1950s, was to identify key variables that might account for successful helping relationships of whatever type, both formal and informal. Rogers (1957) famously postulated that three core conditions—empathy, acceptance, and genuineness (in present-day terminology)—were necessary and sufficient for beneficial helping relationships. Although subsequent findings have qualified Rogers' hypotheses considerably, there is still much interest in the *Rogerian triad* of variables, particularly the concept of empathy (Bohart & Greenberg, 1997).

With the notable exception of Rogers' work, the common factors literature is concerned only with formal helping. Psychotherapy researchers have conducted their studies with little reference to nonprofessional contexts, such as the psychological helping that occurs in everyday settings. It would seem sensible to extend such thinking to a broader range of helping contexts. It is likely that helping in couples will share some common properties with other forms of helping across the spectrum, but it is also highly likely that important differences may exist given the unique nature of couples' relationships.

So, what are the possible core components of psychological helping, and how can we think about these in the context of couples' helping? Process researchers have suggested many different ways of conceptualizing such core components, and different ones may be useful for different purposes (Barker & Pistrang, 2002). Our own preferred conceptualization, which is intended to apply to both formal and informal helping, comprises three broad processes: *establishing a working alliance*, *making meaning*, and *promoting change*. We discuss each of these in turn below.

ESTABLISHING A WORKING ALLIANCE. It is widely recognized that a central component of helping involves the relationship itself between the helper and the helpee. In the formal helping context, this means the client and therapist establishing that they have the prerequisites for working effectively together. This is often referred to as the *working alliance* (Horvath & Luborsky, 1993) and is usually regarded as having three parts. The first is the *bond* between the client and therapist. Rogerian variables, notably therapist empathy and acceptance, form an important part of what is meant by a strong bond. There is a sense of mutual trust in the relationship, and the client feels able to talk freely about whatever is on his or her mind. The second part of the therapeutic alliance is mutual agreement on the goals of therapy: Do client and therapist have similar views of what they are trying to achieve? The third part is agreement on the therapeutic tasks required in order to reach those goals, that is, the actual procedures that the therapist will employ.

How can the concept of the working alliance be applied to couples' helping? It is important to state at the outset that there are many important differences between client–therapist interactions and partners' interactions. Obvious differences are that partner helping takes place within an existing, broader relationship and that partners have not (usually) received any training in providing psychological help. However, we would argue that processes similar to the working alliance must be present if the relationship is to provide effective help. For example, empathy, acceptance, and a shared set of goals seem crucial to any successful helping interaction.

Although a couple may function harmoniously in many aspects of their relationship (e.g., companionship, sex, and parenting), the helping aspect of their relationship may pose specific difficulties. For example, as we demonstrate later in this chapter, it may be hard, for a multitude of reasons, for a partner to empathize with and accept his or her spouse's concerns, and this may inhibit the spouse from freely expressing his or her feelings. Similarly, each member of the couple may have very different ideas about what kind of help is appropriate or desired in dealing with stresses in their lives.

MAKING MEANING. The second core component of psychological helping consists of the activity of meaning making (Brewin & Power, 1999), that is, making sense of the problem and exploring new ways to think about it. This component particularly comes to the fore in humanistic and psychodynamic approaches to formal helping, which are based on helping clients to come to a better understanding of themselves and their feelings, often exploring how their previous life experiences relate to current problems. The therapist may use exploratory questions, or in the case of psychodynamic therapies in particular, make interpretations designed to bring about insight.

Whereas counselors and therapists often draw on psychological theory in order to understand their clients' problems, informal helpers are usually drawing from a different knowledge base. They tend to use their own life knowledge, their understanding of other people who have faced similar problems (possibly drawn from books, films, or television), and general lay theories of stress.

In the couples context, gaining a new understanding of the problem (or of oneself) may not always be a goal of the helping process. However, in discussing a problem together, a couple may jointly explore its meaning and together make sense of it. Thus a process of coconstructing meaning may occur. Sometimes, the partner may try to provide a new perspective on the problem, and if successful, such efforts may result in the helpee's seeing the difficulty in a new light. Unlike formal helpers, partners are in a unique position, in that they have an inside knowledge of the person and of the difficulty being faced; sometimes, however, this inside knowledge may make it more difficult to help, as it may be hard to step back and see the problem in an impartial way.

PROMOTING CHANGE. The third core component, promoting change, consists of active attempts to change the helpee's thoughts or behavior, for example, by engaging in problem solving or giving advice. This is manifested in particular in cognitive and behavioral approaches to formal helping; psychodynamic and client-centered approaches to therapy tend to de-emphasize this, expecting clients to find their own ways of bringing about change once they have developed sufficient understanding of the problem.

Studies of informal helping suggest that efforts to promote change (in particular, giving advice) occur with high frequency, although such advice is not always welcome or effective (Barker & Lemle, 1987; Knowles, 1979; Pistrang & Barker, 1998). Our own research suggests that partners sometimes experience dilemmas about when and whether to engage in efforts to promote change. For example, a dilemma sometimes experienced by partners of people who are depressed is whether to encourage their depressed spouse to be more active as a way of combating the depression (Harris et al., 2004).

Working Models of Helping

We assume that each helper and helpee will have a *working model* of what good helping consists of and that these models can be mapped onto the core components of helping that we have described above. For trained therapists or counselors, the working model is usually an explicit, theoretical framework. As we have already mentioned, different therapeutic approaches emphasize different components of the helping process.

In contrast, for informal helpers, working models of helping are more likely to be implicit and less well articulated. Theorists and researchers have suggested that couples have lay theories, or broad cognitive schemas, about their relationship that organize and affect marital functioning (Bradbury et al., 2000). Our own data suggest that couples also hold more specific lay theories about the helping aspect of their relationship, that is, what sort of help they expect to receive from or provide to their partner. For example, they may conceptualize helping as allowing their partner to *get things off her chest* or about finding a solution to the problem. Such working models, although usually implicit, can be articulated if partners are encouraged to reflect on their helping interactions.

One way in which working models of helping may become salient is when things go wrong in the helping relationship. Our data suggest that unsuccessful helping often occurs because partners hold disparate working models or assumptions. For example, the helpee may be looking for an opportunity to talk through some difficult or distressing feelings, whereas the helper may be assuming that coming up with useful solutions is required. For a variety of reasons, the couple may never explicitly talk about these clashes of assumptions, and some couples can continue in the same pattern of mutually unsatisfying conversations for many long years.

Summary

In this section, we have described some of the concepts used by process researchers in the psychotherapy and counseling fields and argued that these concepts can be usefully extended to the study of informal helping interactions. Having examined the conceptual background of our approach to couples' helping interactions, we now address some methodological issues. How can researchers go about examining the complex processes of helping that occur between partners in close relationships?

A Method for Studying Couples' Helping Interactions

The method to be described has several distinctive features: a microlevel unit of analysis, an idiographic approach, and the use of qualitative methods. We address each of these in turn.

Microlevel of Analysis

Helping processes in general may be studied at several temporal levels of analysis, ranging from the macrolevel of the enduring characteristics of the couples' helping relationship, through the intermediate level of characteristics of a single helping conversation, down to the microlevel of partners' single responses within that conversation (Goodman & Dooley, 1976).

Much of our own recent work has focused on the response level of analysis. We aim to elucidate some of the complex moment-by-moment processes that occur in couples' helping interactions and thereby provide knowledge that might serve as a basis for interventions designed to help couples communicate more effectively in times of stress.

Our general approach to research is one of methodological pluralism. We consider that different research methods and traditions each have their value in approaching different problems (Barker, Pistrang, & Elliott, 2002). In studying processes at the response level, we have found an idiographic, qualitative approach involving the tape-assisted recall method has proved fruitful.

Idiographic Approaches

Idiographic approaches, focusing in depth on a single individual, have been relatively neglected in psychological research, at least that conducted in North America. The prevailing approach is to study groups of individuals in order to try to establish between-group differences or within-group correlations that can be further generalized. One famous countervailing voice was that of Gordon Allport, who pleaded the case for idiographic approaches: "Instead of growing impatient with the single case and hastening on to generalization, why should we not grow impatient with our generalizations and hasten to the internal pattern?" (Allport, 1962, p. 407). Following Allport's position, we hope to elucidate the internal pattern of couples' helping interactions.

The aim of idiographic research is exploratory and hypothesis generating as opposed to the confirmatory, hypothesis-testing aim of traditional research. The research goal is to provide understanding of the particular case, rather than, at least at this stage, to produce general explanatory models. A detailed understanding, sometimes known as "thick description" (Geertz, 1973), is the ultimate aim: Prediction and generalization are not attempted within this genre of research. Although idiographic research can be done within the quantitative tradition, it is in many ways more compatible with qualitative methods, and it this latter tradition that we follow.

Qualitative Methods

One of the advantages of qualitative methods is that they allow access to individuals' idiosyncratic personal meanings and interpretations. Semistructured interview methods enable the researcher to study in depth the person's thoughts and feelings about, in this case, the communication with his or her partner; these interviews can be combined with observation of specific interactions.

We employ a method known as tape-assisted recall, formerly known as interpersonal process recall (Elliott, 1986). Its essence is to record an interaction and then subsequently to play it back to one or both of the participants. The recording can be stopped at salient points in order for the researcher to inquire about the participants' reactions to the conversation at that particular moment. Both the intention behind a helper's response and also the impact of the response on the helpee can be examined. The main applications of the method so far have been in psychotherapy and counseling interviews, but it has also been used in medical settings and to study informal helping. Tape-assisted recall is usually done within a qualitative, phenomenological framework, although the method is also quite compatible with quantitative approaches; for example, participants can rate responses on selected variables such as empathy or helpfulness.

The main advantages of the tape-assisted recall method are that (a) it enables microlevel analysis of specific conversations, because it focuses on a detailed, moment-by-moment account, often seeking the participants' reactions to each talking turn; (b) it integrates observational data (the recording of the interaction) with self-report data (the participants' phenomenological accounts from the recall interview); and (c) it enables the perspective of both participants in an interaction to be compared (partners in a couple can be interviewed either jointly or separately).

In the following sections, we present two case examples from our research in which we took an idiographic approach using the tape-assisted recall method. The examples are intended to illustrate the richness of the data that can be obtained from such methods and the complexity of couples' thoughts and feelings about the process of psychological helping within their relationship.

Case Example 1: Talking About Breast Cancer

The Study

Our first case example comes from an intensive study of four married couples in which the women had recently been treated for breast cancer (Pistrang et al., 1997). Each couple first participated in a semistructured helping conversation. This consisted of a 15-minute audiotaped interaction in which the wife (referred to as the discloser) was asked to talk about a personal concern having to do with her illness and the husband (the helper) was asked to try to be helpful in whatever way seemed natural to him. After the conversation, the partners participated in parallel tape-assisted recall sessions (i.e., the tape-assisted recall sessions were conducted separately with the wife and husband). This procedure consisted of playing back the audiotape of the conversation and stopping after each talking turn to ask a standard series of questions. The questions focused on two key dimensions: the impact of the helper's response on the discloser and the intention behind the helper's response.

Mr. and Mrs. B were in their late 30s and had been married for 14 years; they had three school-age children. Mr. B worked as an administrator in a sales department, and Mrs. B worked as a part-time secretary. Mrs. B had been diagnosed with breast cancer 16 months ago and had been treated by lumpectomy, radiotherapy, and chemotherapy. Mrs. B had an extensive family history of breast cancer.

The Conversation and the Tape-Assisted Recall

In the first part of the conversation, Mrs. B talked about her fear of the cancer recurring. The following episode begins approximately 30 seconds into the conversation. Numbers refer to the talking turn and the letters D or H indicate whether the discloser (woman) or the helper (man) is speaking.[1]

---

[1]The transcription uses a simple notation so as not to impede its readability. Square brackets indicate fragmentary interruptions or editorial insertions. Three dots are used to denote editorial omissions within a talking turn or a trailing off by the speaker at the end of a talking turn.

5 D: I think probably if it came back then I'd have to have more, even if it was still very small, that they would give me more treatment [H: More radium?] [D: Yeah.] [H: I think so, yeah] to try and stop it coming back again and uh, also the chemotherapy. I don't really like injections and things anyway, so, it's not particularly nice. It's quite lucky I wasn't sick or anything the first time but . . .

6 H: Yeah, with a bit of good luck and good fortune smiling upon you, you hopefully won't have a recurrence. [D: No, but . . .] I mean your mum, well your mum's had a mastectomy, but your mum hasn't had any problems at all has she?

7 D: I think the mastectomy is different, I mean [H: Yeah.] and she had such extensive treatment, her treatment was for a year that they probably just killed off anything and everything anyway . . .

In the tape-assisted recall session, Mrs. B said that she felt her husband meant well, but that there was a clash between their styles of coping:

Because I know [partner], I know he's being as supportive and as helpful as he sees that he can, but often he is very flip about life, it's just the way he is. He doesn't allow for anything to worry him, until it happens, and then he worries about it. I sometimes get a bit angry with him, I know he means well, but it's not exactly what you want. You know it's not purposeful, it's just his character.

She also felt irritated with his comparison of her mother with herself:

You can't liken what my mother had and me. Our diagnostics and operations were miles apart, also years apart . . . It [his response] didn't seem to have any real input to the particular problem, the thing I was talking about—recurrence in myself. It was the wrong response.

She felt his intention was "to try to lighten it up, make it less serious." She would have liked him to

. . . make more positive sounds, like "Yes, it may come back, but we're here, we'll get through it." Something more supportive than just "No, we won't worry about that 'til it happens"—because sometimes you do need to worry about it, so that you're prepared. It's doing that "brushing it under the carpet" thing, "just ignore it and it'll go away"—I don't think you can.

Mr. B said his intention was to "try to put her thoughts onto a positive line, always look on the bright side of things, always be optimistic rather than pessimistic." He did not feel that anything got in the way of his being helpful at this point. He noted that *he* felt better for reassuring his wife that things were going to be okay.

This brief interchange (Turns 5–7) encapsulates a discrepancy between the partners' styles of coping with emotional distress and their working models, or beliefs, about how to be helpful. Mr. B attempts to reassure and be upbeat: His message is "look on the bright side." Although Mrs. B recognizes her husband's good intentions, his response fails to acknowledge her fears of recurrence. This does not get addressed directly in the conversation but emerges clearly in the tape-assisted recall.

This same theme and variants of it recur throughout much of the conversation. In the excerpt below, Mrs. B had begun to talk about how to deal with the fear and her need to express her distress.

15 D: Yeah, um, it's just difficult. It's difficult to even know what it is that does frighten you sometimes. And sometimes you just want to sit down and have a real good cry. And, you're not really sure why it is that you want to have a real good cry. I think I've had lots more bouts of lows since the diagnostics and the operation, etc., than I ever had before. I mean I was usually quite uppy, quite often get low and depressed and . . .

16 H: Well I think that it's natural, I mean you're pretty bouncy most of the time. It's rare you get a real downer, very rare.

17 D: That's because I feel that I have to be. Sometimes you're sort of pressurizing yourself into behavior that maybe you don't, you don't really feel like you want to be at this party but here you are anyway so you just make the best time of it. I mean you're treating life in the same fashion; "I'm here, let's just get on and enjoy it," but inside, you're thinking "this is just . . ."

18 H: Yeah, but if you let the inside take over, it's a downward spiral, isn't it? You've got to keep on top of it, you've got to. I mean you've done well up until now, keeping on top of it.

19 D: Sometimes you just want to let go. I mean you help me to stay up on top, but I don't know, sometimes maybe it's not a bad thing to kind of let go and . . .

20 H: Oh it's always a good thing to have a good howl and a cry and tell someone how you feel, but um . . .

21 D: It's embarrassing too. I mean, you feel that you're upsetting the people around you and somehow letting them down. I mean, I couldn't howl in front of the children.

Mr. B's responses at Turns 16 and 18 again illustrate his attitude of being positive: He emphasizes the importance of keeping negative emotions at bay. At Turn 20, he does acknowledge that expressing feelings may be helpful. However, he ends this acknowledgment with a *but*, which seems to express an ambivalence about the usefulness of expressing feelings: The *but* seems to partially retract the acknowledgment. Following this, at Turn 21, Mrs. B hints at her own ambivalence about expressing painful feelings. This is more explicit in the tape-assisted recall in which she described both wanting her husband to give her "permission to let go," as well as her own reluctance to do this (and her envy of others who do): "I've built up a wall where I don't allow emotions out, so it annoys me when others dare to."

Examining the conversation as it evolved over time, we identified a cyclical process in the interaction with a periodicity of about 10 talking turns that revolved around the couple's ambivalences about disclosing painful emotions. In each cycle, Mrs. B expresses her need to "let feelings out," and Mr. B focuses on being positive and the hazards of letting feelings out; Mrs. B then concurs with this view but soon afterward comes back to her need to "let go." The conversation seems like a dance around the core issue—the fear of expressing painful feelings—that never gets talked about directly or resolved.

Summary

Mr. B's attempts to be helpful were clearly well-intentioned, but they often did not match up with Mrs. B's needs and therefore did not have a beneficial impact. Interestingly, this intention–impact discrepancy was not explicitly discussed in the conversation itself, nor was it apparent from quantitative measures that we also included in the study. (Mrs. B tended to rate Mr. B as very supportive and understanding.) It was only in the tape-assisted recall sessions, in which detailed questions were asked about each participant's experience of the conversation, that the personal meanings of the interaction in the context of the couple's relationship became clear.

Mr. and Mrs. B each had their own characteristic, but discrepant, ways of coping with stress. Consistent with these styles of coping, they also seemed to have different working models of helping, that is, what they each assumed was needed in providing help within the relationship. Mrs. B felt that it was important to prepare for potential problems (in this case, a recurrence of cancer) and thus wanted an opportunity to talk about this with her husband and express her distress (although she also expressed ambivalence about this). In contrast, Mr. B's coping style was to take an optimistic stance and not think about potential problems until they occurred; his approach to helping reflected this coping style and thus failed to recognize his wife's needs.

Mr. B's approach to helping may have been shaped by a number of factors, including the painfulness of talking about a possible recurrence of cancer. As he himself noted, his effort to help his wife "look on the bright side" made him feel better; thus, his helping strategy may have been motivated, in part, by a need to reduce his own distress (Coyne et al., 1990). It is interesting to note that Mr. B also mentioned later in the tape-assisted recall interview that he had previously experienced a period of depression following an operation and what he had learned from that was the importance of being positive. He thus seemed to be drawing on his own personal experience in his efforts to support his wife. What he did not seem to realize, however, was that his own beliefs and assumptions about coping and his working model of helping were discrepant from hers.

Case Example 2: The Communication of Empathy in the Transition to Parenthood

Our second case example is drawn from a study of how empathy is communicated in the helping interactions of couples expecting their first baby (Pistrang, Picciotto, & Barker, 2001).

Empathy can be defined as being able to see the world as the other person sees it (Bohart & Greenberg, 1997; see also chap. 4, this volume). It is a necessary condition for engaging in psychological helping interactions (or social interactions of any kind); if a person does not understand the other person's current feelings and state of mind, little effective interaction is likely to result. Our own research suggests that empathy may be an important, although potentially problematic, aspect of psychological helping in couples (Barker & Lemle, 1987; Pistrang & Barker, 1995, 1998). Partners may find it hard to set aside their own feelings or perspective about a concern that affects both members of the couple, compared to an outsider who is somewhat removed from the situation.

The role of empathy in psychotherapy and counseling has aroused interest ever since Rogers' (1957) assertion that it was one of the necessary and sufficient conditions for therapeutic change. As we noted earlier in this chapter, empathy has been identified as one of the factors defining the quality of the working alliance, which in turn is one of the best predictors of successful outcome in therapy (Horvath & Luborsky, 1993). In addition, many authors (including ourselves) believe that empathy has a more direct mechanism for effecting change: In Bohart and Greenberg's (1997, p. 5) words, empathy is "a major component of the healing process." The empathic process, in which one person attempts to understand the other's world and put the understanding into words, can lead to greater self-understanding and self-acceptance in the other (Bohart & Greenberg; Jordan, 1997; Rogers, 1975).

Despite the recognition that empathy plays an important role in psychological helping, little is known about how it is communicated. What does the helper do that leads to the helpee feeling understood? Recent research in counseling and psychotherapy suggests that empathy, as experienced by the client, does not seem to have a simple correspondence to specific therapist responses. The therapist's understanding of and intention to understand the client may be conveyed through patterns of interactions that vary with context and perspective (Bohart & Tallman, 1997). It is likely that the same is true in informal helping interactions, although we can only make conjectures because of the paucity of research focusing on empathy in informal helping.

The Study

The study aimed to provide a detailed description of how empathy is communicated and experienced in couples about to become parents for the first time. The transition to parenthood, although not generally experienced as a crisis event, is often a stressful time in the family life cycle (Cowan & Cowan, 1999). Each member of the couple may have concerns about new roles and responsibilities, and being able to talk about and help each other with such concerns would seem to be an important part of the process of adaptation.

A total of 18 couples, all expecting their first baby, participated in the study. Each couple participated in a semistructured helping conversation similar to that described in the first case example. The woman (the discloser) was asked to talk about a personal concern related to the transition to parenthood, and the man (the helper) was asked to try to be helpful in whatever way seemed natural. The couple then participated in a joint tape-assisted recall session, in contrast to our earlier example in which the tape-assisted recall sessions were conducted separately. The first stage of the tape-assisted recall procedure involved identifying helper responses that were high and low in empathy: Each member of the couple independently rated each helper response on a scale of empathy. The second stage involved selecting a sample of high- and low-empathy responses from the discloser's ratings and then discussing these in detail using a semi-structured interview. The discussion focused on each partner's experience of those specific moments in the conversation, for example, what it was about the helper's response that made the discloser feel understood (or not) and what it was the helper was trying to do at that particular point.

Natalie and Neil were in their early 30s and had been living together for 4 years. Both worked in the public relations field. Natalie was 8 months pregnant at the time of the study. In the semistructured helping conversation, Natalie chose to talk about her concern that her identity might change after the baby was born. As she put it: "[I'm concerned about] becoming less Natalie and becoming a mother to a child, as well as being Natalie, as well as being Neil's Natalie, and everybody else's Natalie. And I just see it as Natalie being a whole and then bits taken away from it." Below we present two episodes from the conversation, each of which contains one low-empathy and one high-empathy response as perceived by the discloser. Each excerpt is followed by material from the tape-assisted recall session.

EPISODE 1. The following episode begins approximately 3 minutes into the conversation. The low-empathy response is indicated by one asterisk, and the high-empathy response by two asterisks.

14 H:　 . . . when you said . . . you can't keep everybody happy all the time, you just have to piss everybody off a little bit, what that's about is like sort of evening it about a bit really isn't it? It's not about, so [D: Yeah, but what about the Natalie bit?] everybody gives a bit don't they?

15 D:　 I'm just worried about the Natalie bit.

16 H:*　 But isn't that, I mean there isn't, you're not really talking about Natalie on her own are you? You're talking about Natalie with her friends or Natalie in different situations.

17 D:　 No, I'm, I'm talking about Natalie on her own, the individual [H: Are you?] the person, the me, the thinking time for me [H: Yeah, right] on my own.

18 H:**　 Well everyone needs that.

19 D:　 Well yeah, but when do you get it, when you've got a baby?

20 H:　 I don't know, actually (both laugh). I'm not sure . . .

In the tape-assisted recall session, Natalie rated Neil's response at Turn 16 as low in empathy. She felt he had made an inaccurate interpretation of what she had been saying:

> I felt that he was interpreting what I said rather than listening to what I said . . . and that wasn't what I'd been talking about so I didn't feel like he'd listened at all, basically . . . was the words he chose, I think. He said, "You're not talking about this, you're talking about that," and that to me sounded really kind of, "I'm telling you what you're saying," rather than "I've listened and I think what you're saying is . . ."

Neil, on the other hand, said that his intention was to try to clarify what Natalie was concerned about:

> It wasn't intended as an "I'm telling you," it was trying to clarify really, for me. I think in order to get to empathy you need to clarify your understanding of things. You can't just have empathy. If I can clarify it for myself, then that puts me in a better position to be able to react to it, understand it and therefore be more helpful. But maybe it was a bit quick.

Natalie would have liked Neil to have been more tentative:

I just think using different terminology, saying "You know, I think that what you're trying to say is . . .," or "I felt that what you're trying to say is . . .," rather than "You're trying to say this." That would have made me feel better. It was being told that that was what I was thinking that was the problem.

In contrast, Natalie experienced Neil's next response at Turn 18 as high in empathy because it acknowledged the essence of her concern. She described its impact in the following way:

. . . saying "well everyone needs that" was kind of like manna from heaven. . . . It was acknowledging something that we don't really talk about, the fact that everyone needs time to think, and time on their own. We have had rows about it, we've talked about it before, so when he said that it was like, fantastic . . . [His response] could be interpreted as a bit dismissive in some ways couldn't it? But because [he's] never ever said that before, that's a very rare thing for him to say, to acknowledge that everyone needs thinking time.

For his part, Neil felt that he had understood what the issue was:

I did know what she was talking about, it's a topic that has been discussed in other contexts. It's not something that I would have always said in that situation, but more recently in our relationship it's something that would come up naturally, it's something that I have a better understanding of.

EPISODE 2. The next episode occurred approximately two minutes later in the conversation. The couple had been talking about ways in which Natalie might find time away from the baby and how Neil would look after the baby at those times. At this point, Natalie had begun to talk about her feeling that she would have ultimate responsibility for the baby. Again, the low- and high-empathy responses are marked by one and two asterisks, respectively.

31 D: Yeah, yeah, but I know, but it's different, isn't it, because the woman just automatically feels that the ultimate responsibility—it's what [my sister] was saying to me, the ultimate responsibility for the child rests with the woman, or she feels it rests with her [H: Right]. It's like you are the default, as the woman you are the default, if the man can't make it home on time from work you have to be there, there's no choice there.

32 H:* Yeah, but that's rather dependent upon the man as well isn't it [D: Well yeah, it is . . .] and on the type of man (laugh) [D: It is] and I think that's a poor example to give.

33 D: Well, all right, well you need to prove it different.

34 H: . . . yeah all right, but you haven't given me a chance to prove it otherwise, all I'm saying is that if you want to sort of have things that you do, like if you want to do your drama or something, then you could do it, couldn't you? . . . it's not a problem, you should have interests outside of the house anyway, shouldn't you?

35 D: Yep.

36 H: Yeah? Have you thought what you'd do?

37 D: No, but I'd probably want to do something that doesn't involve interface, 'cause that's the whole point.

38 H: Like what (laughs), sitting on your arse reading a book?

39 D: Yeah, probably! Something like that, because that's the whole point . . . I get tired at work of interfacing and talking to clients and all that [H: Yeah] and then coming home and having to entertain the baby and entertain you and all that sort of thing, so sometimes that's exactly what I want [H: (laughs) Entertain me!], is a morning where I can just sit on my arse reading a book and get completely lost in it [H: Yeah] . . . and don't have to worry about, you know, where things are or doing anything at all, just have completely selfish time.

40 H: Well, I know.

41 D: But doing drama wouldn't be like that.

42 H:** Right, okay. So are you worried, so, uh, don't know, are you worried that outwardly it would just look lazy or something? Cause I accept that this is, that you need to have time for yourself [D: Do you?], that you kind of like spread the things out.

43 D: Do you?

44 H: Yes.

In the tape-assisted recall session, Natalie rated Neil's response at Turn 32 as low in empathy. She experienced Neil as dismissing her concern:

... I used my sister as an example because she'd talked about that—the fact that she feels all the time that it boils down to her, but then I'd taken that beyond that. I'd said that generally I think it defaults to the woman to have the responsibility, and then Neil, I felt, was quite dismissive because he was saying "I know who we're talking about and I'm not going to be like that." He was dismissing my generalization.

Neil explained that his response was partly motivated by self-defense:

I focused more on the [brother-in-law] thing, and not wanting to be bagged up with someone I don't consider myself in the same bag as. I kind of felt that you'd insulted me almost by bagging me up with somebody that you've dismissed as well as I have, so I felt that I had to sort of say "Come on, don't do that."

However, his intention was also to reassure Natalie:

In a way [I was] trying to be reassuring, trying to say that not everyone is like that, not just from a defensive point of view, but also from a "don't just expect the worst from everybody, other people can be different." So in a way I was dismissive of the frame of reference, but it was because I was saying "there is something else that's a possibility there."

Following this low-empathy helper response, the conversation resumed its earlier focus on the types of outside interests that Natalie might pursue. This led to Natalie's stating that she didn't really want activities involving *interfacing* with other people, but simply *selfish* time on her own. In the tape-assisted recall session, she rated Neil's next response, at Turn 42, as high in empathy. She described how the response sounded to her, and why:

It was the first time in a long while that he sounded like he was trying to explore what I meant rather than either giving me a solution or tell me what he thought I meant . . . Sounded more exploratory and open, basically. It was the way he started off "So, are you worried about . . .?" sounded like he was really interested in what I was trying to say, rather than the solutionizing that had come before. Or the defensiveness.

Natalie added that Neil's question was actually not an accurate reflection of her concern, but she experienced it as empathic nonetheless:

That wasn't right, actually, that it would just look lazy, but he was asking me, rather than saying "You're thinking this," and then being really reassuring after that saying "It's acceptable." So it was a reassuring note along with an inquiring note I think.

She felt it was an important moment in the conversation, in that she and Neil were finally coming back to her central concern. As she put it: "I think we almost went back to the beginning of the conversation where we were beginning to explore."

Neil said that his intention at that point was to check his understanding of what Natalie had been saying:

I felt that there was a bit of realization for me . . . I felt like I'd got to another level in terms of my understanding of her perspective on this. So what I was trying to do was really just ask a kind of straightforward situation question to see if what I'd understood was right.

For Neil, as well, this was a pivotal moment in the conversation:

That was an important point for me. Up until then I'd been trying to explore, "What do you want to do that will make you happy, what is this event that you need to create?" But then I realized that actually, no, it might just be quite inward, it might not be an outward activity that Natalie needs to be doing, it might be quite fulfilling for it to be inward in a way. That was a movement on.

Summary

The qualitative data from the tape-assisted recall interview suggested that empathy can be communicated within a couple's relationship in a variety of ways, some of which may not be readily apparent to the outside observer. The data also illustrate how things can go wrong in terms of the helpee experiencing a lack of empathy despite good intentions on the part of the helper.

The high-empathy responses illustrated in the excerpts above had several interesting features. The first response, at Turn 18, was experienced by Natalie as an acknowledgment of her concern: She felt that Neil had recognized and accepted her need for "thinking time on my own." Although to an outside observer it might have seemed dismissive (as Natalie herself noted), Neil's acknowledgment was particularly important in the context of their relationship: They previously had arguments about this topic. The second high-empathy response, at Turn 42, was interesting in that Natalie reported that Neil had not actually understood her concern: What was important for her was that he was trying to explore what she meant. Thus, it was the exploratory nature of his question, rather than its accuracy, that felt empathic.

A striking aspect of the low-empathy responses was the discrepancy between the helper's intention and the impact of his response. For example, at Turn 16, Neil's intention was to try to clarify what Natalie was concerned about; however, she felt he was interpreting, rather than listening to, what she had said. (Natalie contrasted this response to the later one at Turn 42, at which point Neil also misunderstood but was more tentative in his attempt to clarify.) The other low-empathy response, at Turn 32, was partly motivated by Neil's need to defend himself but was also intended as reassurance; its effect on Natalie, however, was to feel dismissed rather than reassured.

Although the study did not directly set out to examine the helpfulness of high- and low-empathy responses, the data—both from this case example as well as the larger study from which it is drawn—provide some clues about their different impacts. Low-empathy responses often seemed to impede the development of the conversation and interfere with the process of helping. For example, following the low-empathy response at Turn 32, the couple came close to having an argument about Neil's future role as a father. Natalie (and other participants in the study) described feeling annoyed when she experienced her partner as either dismissing her concern or not listening. The immediate impact of this was often to divert the discloser from talking about her concern or to repeat what she had previously said.

In contrast, high-empathy responses were usually experienced as helpful, indeed, as Natalie described it, like "manna from heaven." Such responses seemed to allow or encourage the discloser to talk more about what she felt. This was particularly evident in Neil's response at Turn 42, which both Natalie and Neil experienced as an important point in the conversation. Natalie felt that Neil's effort to explore what she meant allowed her to get back to the essence of her concern. For his part, Neil felt that he had come to a new understanding of what Natalie was worried about: Prior to this point he had been focusing the conversation on finding activities that would allow Natalie time away from the baby, but he now realized that this was not the central issue. As Natalie put it, they finally seemed to be returning to the start of the conversation after several detours. This was a significant turning point in that both partners now felt they could begin to talk about the real issue, that of how parenthood might have an impact on Natalie's sense of identity.

Implications for Interventions

Something that has struck us as researchers is how often our participants indicate that taking part in the research is in itself a therapeutic experience. In participating in a study, couples typically spend an hour and a half examining their helping communication in close detail. They often say that this experience causes them to think and talk about their communication in a way that they have never done before. By this, they seem to mean that they talk about their helping communication in a detailed way, with a neutral facilitator, in a semistructured procedure, and using a psychological framework. This experience allows them to articulate their experience of helping and being helped, often for the first time, and they emerge with a sense of increased mutual understanding and acceptance.

The research procedures we have used—the semistructured helping conversation and the tape-assisted recall interview—would thus seem to have therapeutic applications. Similar communication tasks in which one partner takes the role of helper and the other as helpee have been used previously in couple interventions (e.g., Guerney, 1977). Although such structured conversations obviously introduce an element of artificiality (because one-way helping rarely occurs in this sort of extended way), they allow a clearer focus on partners' helping styles. Used in conjunction with this type of conversation, the tape-assisted recall procedure then provides a forum in which couples can reflect on the patterns or significant aspects of their interactions. In this way, the tape-assisted recall procedure encourages metacommunication, that is, it can be used to help couples communicate more effectively about their own communication.

Such procedures could be incorporated into interventions targeted at couples facing stresses in their lives. Most of the couple therapy literature focuses on reducing conflict, to the relative neglect of enhancing the helping aspects of couples' relationships. However, recent evidence suggests that supportive interactions may be at least as important as conflictual ones in predicting marital outcomes (Pasch & Bradbury, 1998). Consistent with this, some researchers have proposed that supportive and stressful aspects of relationships are likely to be different processes that coexist (Burman & Margolin, 1992). Although couples facing difficult circumstances or life transitions are at increased risk for experiencing marital distress (e.g., Belsky, 1990; Walker, Johnson, Manion, & Cloutier, 1996), we would speculate that having a strong helping relationship may not only reduce the likelihood of conflict but also increase couples' psychological resources in dealing with problems.

Conclusion

Clearly, the line of research reported here is in its early stages of development and raises a number of issues that we have not addressed in this chapter. Our two case examples both involved the woman as the discloser and the man as the helper. Possible gender differences in helping interactions therefore could not be examined; nor do we mean to imply that women have greater needs for support or that the difficulties in providing appropriate support occur for men only. Our case examples also involved common dyadic stressors (see chap. 2, this volume): Both breast cancer and the transition to parenthood have an impact on the couple, not just on the individual. Whether helping processes differ for different stressors is an area for further research. Finally, the use of tape-assisted recall raises potential validity problems, which we have not addressed (see Elliott, 1986). However, despite these limitations, we hope that our process analysis approach contains a possible way forward for understanding and enhancing the ways in which partners communicate at times of stress.

Our central argument is that is important to examine partners' process of communication as it unfolds from moment to moment and also to examine partners' moment-by-moment perceptions of and reactions to that communication process. We have also proposed some core components of helping relationships that provide a framework for making sense of couples' helping interactions: establishing a working alliance, making meaning, and promoting change. The process analysis approach that we have advocated allows researchers to examine in detail these core components of helping interactions, and thus, has the potential to enrich our understanding of how and when partners' helping efforts are effective or not. For instance, in our first case example, the husband's "look-on-the-bright-side" approach to helping illustrates an unsuccessful attempt to promote change (in his wife's outlook on her illness); this communication was not perceived as helpful by his wife because she wanted some acknowledgment of her fears rather than a change of outlook. In our second case example, one of the key positive moments in the conversation centered on the process of making meaning; interestingly, it was more a process of joint meaning for the couple, rather than for one individual alone. Such examples provide a starting point for developing a more fine-grained understanding of the helping process. Further research is needed, however, to determine whether our proposed core components of helping serve as a useful conceptual framework and descriptive tool.

We have also suggested that partners' perceptions of and reactions to their interactions are partly determined by their preexisting beliefs about what constitutes good helping, which we have labeled *working models of helping*. Such working models are largely implicit, but they can often be inferred from partners' accounts of their communication process. As can be observed from our two case examples, instances when communication is not working optimally are often indicative of disparate agendas being pursued by each partner. Such moments, which have similarities to what psychotherapy researchers describe as "ruptures" in the therapeutic relationship (Safran, 1993), can severely impede the helping process.

A key task for future research is to gain a better understanding of couples' working models of helping. One potentially fruitful approach would be to study "significant events," that is, moments when the helping communication is going particularly well or badly (Rice & Greenberg, 1984). Our own data suggest that negative events (when things are going wrong) provide particularly valuable inroads to understanding partners' working models. Our experience is that it is difficult for couples to articulate their expectations and assumptions about helping in the abstract, but that they can begin to articulate these when listening to recordings of their own interactions. Thus, the tape-assisted recall procedure, which we have described in this chapter, could be used to examine significant events in couples' interactions with the specific aim of elucidating their assumptions about helping and being helped. Whether and how couples' working models map onto the core components of the helping process (e.g., whether they view helping primarily as an effort to promote change or as providing an opportunity to express one's feelings) might also be addressed by further research. A longer term task is to establish whether working models of helping have predictive power: For example, does the degree of congruence in partners' working models predict the quality of their helping communication?

Knowledge about the processes that occur in couples' helping interactions has the potential to provide couples with a better understanding of common pitfalls as well as ways of better meeting each other's needs. Like the partners quoted at the start of this chapter, couples often feel lost and confused about how to respond to each other's distress. Ultimately, our aim is to empower people in relationships to deliver mutual psychological help more effectively.

References

Allport, G. W. (1962). The general and the unique in psychological science. *Journal of Personality, 30,* 405–422.

Barker, C., & Lemle, R. (1987). Informal helping in partner and stranger dyads. *Journal of Marriage and the Family, 49,* 541–547.

Barker, C., & Pistrang, N. (2002). Psychotherapy and social support: Integrating research on psychological helping. *Clinical Psychology Review, 22,* 361–379.

Barker, C., Pistrang, N., & Elliott, R. (2002). *Research methods in clinical psychology* (2nd ed.). Chichester, England: Wiley.

Barker, C., Pistrang, N., Shapiro, D. A., & Shaw, I. (1990). Coping and help-seeking in the UK adult population. *British Journal of Clinical Psychology, 29,* 271–285.

Belsky, J. (1990). Children and marriage. In F. D. Fincham & T. N. Bradbury (Eds.), *The psychology of marriage: Basic issues and applications* (pp. 172–200). New York: Guilford Press.

Blood, R. O., & Wolfe, D. M. (1960). *Husbands and wives: The dynamics of married living.* New York: Free Press.

Bohart, A. C., & Greenberg, L. S. (1997). Empathy and psychotherapy: An introductory overview. In A. C. Bohart & L. S. Greenberg (Eds.), *Empathy reconsidered: New directions in psychotherapy* (pp. 3–31). Washington, DC: American Psychological Association.

Bohart, A. C., & Tallman, K. (1997). Empathy and the active client: An integrative, cognitive–experiential approach. In A. C. Bohart & L. S. Greenberg (Eds.), *Empathy reconsidered: New directions in psychotherapy* (pp. 393–415). Washington, DC: American Psychological Association.

Bradbury, T. N., Fincham, F. D., & Beach, S. R. H. (2000). Research on the nature and determinants of marital satisfaction: A decade in review. *Journal of Marriage and the Family, 62,* 964–980.

Brewin, C. R., & Power, M. J. (1999). Integrating psychological therapies: Processes of meaning transformation. *British Journal of Medical Psychology, 72,* 143–157.

Brown, G. W., & Harris, T. (1978). *Social origins of depression: A study of psychiatric disorder in women.* London: Tavistock.

Burleson, B. R., Albrecht, T. L., & Sarason, I. G. (Eds.). (1994). *Communication of social support: Messages, interactions, relationships, and community.* Thousand Oaks, CA: Sage.

Burman, B., & Margolin, G. (1992). Analysis of the association between marital relationships and health problems: An interactional perspective. *Psychological Bulletin, 112,* 39–63.

Christensen, A., & Jacobson, N. S. (1994). Who (or what) can do psychotherapy: The status and challenge of the nonprofessional psychotherapies. *Psychological Science, 5,* 8–14.

Cowan, C. P., & Cowan, P. A. (1999). *When partners become parents: The big life change for couples.* London: Erlbaum.

Cowen, E. (1982). Help is where you find it: Four informal helping groups. *American Psychologist, 37,* 385–395.

Coyne, J. C., & DeLongis, A. (1986). Going beyond social support: The role of social relationships in adaptation. *Journal of Consulting and Clinical Psychology, 54,* 454–460.

Coyne, J. C., Ellard, J. H., & Smith, D. A. F. (1990). Social support, interdependence, and the dilemmas of helping. In B. R. Sarason, I. G. Sarason, & G. R. Pierce (Eds.), *Social support: An interactional view,* (pp. 129–149). New York: Wiley.

Cutrona, C. E. (1996). *Social support in couples.* Thousand Oaks, CA: Sage.

Cutrona, C. E., & Suhr, J. A. (1994). Social support communication in the context of marriage: An analysis of couples' supportive interactions. In B. R. Burleson, T. L. Albrecht, & I. G. Sarason (Eds.), *Communication of social support: Messages, interactions, relationships and community.* Thousand Oaks, CA: Sage.

Dakof, G. A., & Taylor, S. E. (1990). Victims' perceptions of social support: What is helpful from whom? *Journal of Personality and Social Psychology, 58,* 80–89.

Elliott, R. (1986). Interpersonal Process Recall (IPR) as a process research method. In L. Greenberg & W. Pinsof (Eds.), *The psychotherapeutic process: A research handbook* (pp. 503–527). New York: Guilford Press.

Fincham, F. D., & Bradbury, T. N. (1990). Social support in marriage: The role of social cognition. *Journal of Social and Clinical Psychology, 9*, 31–42.

Geertz, C. (1973). *The interpretation of cultures*. New York: Basic Books.

Goodman, G., & Dooley, D. (1976). A framework for help-intended communication. *Psychotherapy: Theory, Research and Practice, 13*, 106–117.

Guerney, B. G. (1977). *Relationship enhancement: Skill-training programs for therapy, problem prevention, and enrichment*. San Francisco: Jossey-Bass.

Harris, T., Pistrang, N., & Barker, C. (2004). *Couples' experiences of the support process in depression: A phenomenological analysis*. Manuscript submitted for publication.

Hogan, B. E., Linden, B. E., & Najarian, B. (2002). Social support interventions: Do they work? *Clinical Psychology Review, 22*, 381–440.

Horvath, A. O., & Luborsky, L. (1993). The role of the therapeutic alliance in psychotherapy. *Journal of Consulting and Clinical Psychology, 61*, 561–573.

Hubble, M. A., Duncan, B. L., & Miller, S. D. (1999). *The heart and soul of change: What works in therapy*. Washington, DC: American Psychological Association.

Jordan, J. V. (1997). A relational perspective for understanding women's development. In J. V. Jordan (Ed.), *Women's growth in diversity: More writings from the Stone Center* (pp. 9–24). New York: Guilford Press.

Knowles, D. (1979). On the tendency for volunteer helpers to give advice. *Journal of Counseling Psychology, 26*, 352–354.

Lanza, A. F., Cameron, A. E., & Revenson, T. A. (1995). Helpful and unhelpful support among individuals with rheumatic diseases. *Psychology & Health, 10*, 449–462.

Lehman, D. R., Ellard, J. H. & Wortman, C. B. (1986). Social support for the bereaved: Recipients' and providers' perspectives on what is helpful. *Journal of Consulting and Clinical Psychology, 54*, 438–446.

Manne, S. L. (1998). Cancer in the marital context: A review of the literature. *Cancer Investigation, 16*, 188–202.

Milne, D. L. (1999). *Social therapy: A guide to social support interventions for mental health practitioners*. New York: Wiley.

Nye, F. I. (1976). *Role structure and analysis of the family*. Beverly Hills, CA: Sage.

Pasch, L. A., & Bradbury, T. N. (1998). Social support, conflict, and the development of marital dysfunction. *Journal of Consulting and Clinical Psychology, 66*, 219–230.

Pistrang, N., & Barker, C. (1995). The partner relationship in psychological response to breast cancer. *Social Science and Medicine, 40*, 789–797.

Pistrang, N., & Barker, C. (1998). Partners and fellow patients: Two sources of emotional support for women with breast cancer. *American Journal of Community Psychology, 26*, 439–456.

Pistrang, N., Barker, C., & Rutter, C. (1997). Social support as conversation: Analysing breast cancer patients' interactions with their partners. *Social Science and Medicine, 45*, 773–782.

Pistrang, N., Picciotto, A., & Barker, C. (2001). The communication of empathy in couples during the transition to parenthood. *Journal of Community Psychology, 29*, 615–636.

Rice, L. N., & Greenberg, L. S. (Eds.). (1984). *Patterns of change: Intensive analysis of psychotherapy process*. New York: Guilford Press.

Rogers, C. R. (1957). The necessary and sufficient conditions of therapeutic personality change. *Journal of Consulting Psychology, 21*, 95–103.

Rogers, C. R. (1975). Empathic: An unappreciated way of being. *The Counseling Psychologist, 5*, 2–10.

Safran, J. D. (1993). The therapeutic alliance rupture as a trans-theoretical phenomenon: Definitional and conceptual issues. *Journal of Psychotherapy Integration, 3*, 33–49.

Sarason, B. R., Sarason, I. G., & Pierce, G. R. (Eds.). (1990). *Social support: An interactional view*. New York: Wiley.

Stiles, W. B., Shapiro, D. A., & Elliott, R. (1986). "Are all psychotherapies equivalent?" *American Psychologist, 41*, 165–180.

Veroff, J., Kulka, R. A., & Douvan, E. (1981). *Mental health in America: Patterns of help-seeking from 1957 to 1976*. New York: Basic Books.

Walker, J. G., Johnson, S. L., Manion, I., & Cloutier, P. (1996). Emotionally focused marital intervention for couples with chronically ill children. *Journal of Consulting and Clinical Psychology, 64*, 1029–1036.

6

My Illness or Our Illness? Attending to the Relationship When One Partner Is Ill

Linda K. Acitelli and Hoda J. Badr

In this chapter, we present a blending of literatures on relationships, gender differences, and chronic illness. Much has been written regarding how relationships affect individuals' health, how chronic illnesses affect individual outcomes, and the gender differences in health outcomes. What is unique to this chapter is its focus on relationship outcomes rather than individual outcomes. One of our aims in this chapter is to further expand the idea that chronic illnesses affect not only the unhealthy individuals but the relationships of these individuals as well. We argue that people need take a relationship perspective when adapting their lives to their own or their partners' chronic illnesses.

When a significant other is ailing, taking a relationship perspective involves seeing the health problem not in individual terms but in relational terms. One way that a relationship perspective is manifested is by discussing the relationship. Earlier research has shown that talking about one's relationship is viewed in different ways by men and women (Acitelli, 1988). These different viewpoints highlight the distinction between routine and strategic relationship maintenance (Dainton & Stafford, 1993). Women view relationship talk as part of everyday relationship functioning (routine maintenance), whereas men value it to the extent that it is used to solve a relationship problem (strategic maintenance). This gender difference has implications for heterosexual couples coping with chronic illness, or any stressor for that matter. Accordingly, husbands and wives may treat illness differently depending on the extent to which they see a spouse's disease as a relationship problem or an individual problem. If both partners take a relationship perspective, they see the illness as a problem for the relationship, rather than just a problem for one individual. They are both more likely to engage in relationship talk as a way to cope and maintain the relationship. Couples who become aware of and discuss the relationship implications of a partner's illness can anticipate how their relationships may change and prepare for the difficulties they may face.

The concept of relationship awareness provides a framework for studying the attending to relationships (e.g., Acitelli, 1992). Relationship awareness is defined as a person's focusing attention on a relationship or on interaction patterns, comparisons, or contrasts between partners in a relationship, including attending to the couple or relationship as an entity. Earlier work has made the important distinction between thinking and talking within the context of a relationship and thinking and talking about the relationship. Cognition and communication may occur within the context of a relationship yet not focus on the relationship per se. For example, one partner may reflect on the other partner's illness by thinking about *how difficult it must be for her* and may even tell her so. The thought and speech are focused on an individual partner within a relationship context but are not focused on the relationship itself. However, if the partner were to think that *her illness affects my life, too,* then the partner is beginning to focus on the relationship because he is acknowledging both partners. He is thinking about something about her that affects him (as opposed to something about her that affects her quality of life). He might even focus more squarely on the relationship by telling her that he sees her difficulties as *our difficulties,* thereby taking a relationship perspective in dealing with her illness. Taking a relationship perspective is a form of relationship awareness.

Next, we define the different forms of relationship awareness and how they can be applied to the illness in the relationship context. In later sections we suggest directions for future studies. Finally, we present our investigations that focus specifically on relationship talk, health, and relationship outcomes.

Implications of Relationship Awareness for Coping With Chronic Illness

In order to examine the possible links between relationship awareness, relationship outcomes, and chronic illness, the concept of relationship awareness must be explained.

Forms of Relationship Awareness

Relationship awareness is a multifaceted concept and manifests itself in different forms. Both thinking and talking in relationship terms are considered ways of attending to the relationship or different forms of relationship awareness. Our work begins to delineate the forms that attention to the relationship can take. Extending the reasoning of Polanyi (1966) and Wegner and Giuliano (1982), we make the distinction between *explicit* relationship awareness and *implicit* relationship awareness, highlighting the difference between *topics of thought* and *perspectives on these topics.* Thus, these two dimensions (explicit vs. implicit relationship awareness and talk vs. thought) can be combined to create four forms of relationship awareness, shown in Figure 6.1.

If the relationship is the focal object of one's attention, then the awareness is explicit. If the relationship is the lens through which one approaches topics of talking or thinking, then relationship awareness is implicit. The approach one takes or the lens one uses to observe the object of explicit awareness would be the subject of one's implicit awareness. One question we ask is, through

	Thinking	Talking
Explicit	A relationship partner reminiscing (worrying) about the good (bad) times they've had together.	"I'm so glad (upset that) we (don't) know how to work on being healthy together."
Implicit	A relationship partner perceiving joys (problems) as relationship (our) joys (problems) no matter what the topic.	"We cope with his illness together" versus "He copes with his illness on his own."

Figure 6.1. Examples of the four forms of relationship awareness.

which lens do partners in relationships look, or what is the subject of their implicit awareness, the self lens or the relationship lens? Wegner and Guiliano (1982) posit that keeping an entity (in this case, the relationship) in implicit awareness helps maintain a positive view of the entity (relationship). Implicit awareness of the relationship makes a negative evaluation of both the relationship and the partner unlikely and helps maintain a positive evaluation of the partner and the relationship.

Implicit thinking in relationship terms means taking a couple orientation toward the world and tending to think of oneself in terms of *we*. For example, a person perceives joys or problems in the relationship as *our* joys or problems. In other words, the person is taking a relationship perspective, similar to a couple identity (Acitelli, Rogers, & Knee, 1999). Implicit awareness is also manifested in speech. For example, if a person is implicitly aware of the relationship and is asked how her ill husband is coping, she might answer, "We cope with his illness together." On the other hand, a person who does not maintain an implicit awareness of the relationship might say, "He copes with his illness on his own."

Explicit thinking in relationship terms involves conscious thought about the relationship. A person focuses on interactions patterns or the differences between partners in the relationship or thinks about the relationship as an entity (e.g., "Our relationship works well"). The emotional tone of the thinking can be positive or negative. For example, a person may reminisce about all the good times they have had together or worry that the partners are not as close as they used to be (Cate, Koval, Lloyd, & Wilson, 1995). Explicit talking about the relationship is similar to explicit thinking, such that the person talks explicitly about the relationship in the same terms that he or she thinks about it, for example, "I'm so glad (or upset) that we (don't) know how to work on being healthy together." Explicit talking is similar to metacommunication when it involves partners talking about their communication patterns or patterns of interaction.

The four forms of relationship awareness are not independent of one another. For example, we assume that when people talk, they have, at some level, thought about it before they speak. Thus, the explicit and implicit forms of talking are not independent of the explicit and implicit forms of thinking. Yet one can think about a relationship without talking about it. So explicit and implicit thinking about the relationship can exist independently of talking, but talking must be preceded by thinking. Explicit forms and implicit forms of relationship awareness may or may not be related to one another. A person may think explicitly about interaction patterns (e.g., "When he is having a bad day, I do more things for him than when he has good days") and subsequently see the partner's illness as a relationship issue rather than one partner's issue. However, a person who thinks explicitly might obsess endlessly about the couples' interaction patterns (e.g., "I get so upset when she is obviously suffering") without actually seeing the illness in *we* terms (implicit awareness). On the other hand, couples can see the illness in *we* terms but never think or talk explicitly about the relationship. This would occur most likely in cultures in which gender roles are well defined. For example, studies have shown that less acculturated Mexican American couples are more religious and traditional in their sex role ideology than are those couples who are more acculturated (Frisbie, Optiz, & Kelly, 1985; Sabogal, Marin, Otero-Sabogal, Marin, & Perez-Stable, 1987). In couples who adopt traditional sex roles, each partner assumes that the other will take on the expected role and relate to the partner in ways that the culture has prescribed for them without talking about it. Thus, there could be less need to talk about the relationship because the culture already defines for them how a relationship is supposed to be.

Our general hypothesis is that it is better for the well-being of a relationship to take a relationship perspective when a partner is ill. That is, couples who see the illness as a relationship issue rather than an individual issue will be more satisfied with their relationship than couples who do not. We are not the first researchers to think about chronic illness in the context of relationships. Coyne for example, has written a great deal on relationship-focused coping (Coyne & Smith, 1991); with his colleagues (Lyons, Sullivan, Ritvo, & Coyne, 1995), he has written about how important it is for friends, relatives, and coworkers to engage in communal coping, whereby it becomes a team effort. The work of Kayser, Sormanti, and Strainchamps (1999) focuses on the influence of relational factors on women coping with cancer. Revenson (1994, 2003, chap. 7, this volume) has developed a congruence model of coping for couples faced with a serious disabling illness and addressed how gender may affect couples' coping. However, most of these studies focus on how well and in what ways partners cope as it relates to an individual's psychological adjustment. Our work focuses on coping and social support as it relates to relationship outcomes, for example, relationship satisfaction or stability.

Four Forms of Relationship Awareness in the Context of Illness

To explain in more detail how these forms of relationship awareness can be applied to couples' coping within the illness context, we apply our conceptualization illustrated in Figure 6.1 to couples in which one person has a chronic illness. Examples from qualitative studies are used to clarify the different forms of relationship awareness and how they relate to relationship outcomes. Then, we present quantitative studies on one form, explicit relationship talk, as it relates to health and relationship outcomes

We use case examples of implicit talking, explicit talking, explicit thinking, and implicit thinking to illustrate the four forms of relationship awareness. Our first example illustrates how conflict can occur if neither partner takes a relationship perspective. We have taken the examples from published qualitative studies by other researchers in which one partner has a serious or chronic illness.

This first example, from a sociological study of the self in chronic illness (Charmaz, 1991, p. 172) shows what can occur if spouses view the illness as an individual's problem. Neither of them seem to think or talk in relationships terms.

> A middle-aged man had convalesced for several months when his wife began to push him to go back to work. He remarked, "My wife put it to me one day; she said, in one of her less charitable moments . . . 'What are you going to do today? Well, what are you going to do today? Recover?' And I went and I thought and said, 'What I'm going to do today is try to live my life without reacting to structures that I can't meet [or] cope with anyway.' And that's basically the whole philosophy of life I guess I am approaching the world with these days. At least to the extent I can. And it's really severely important to me—to not live my life according to somebody else's, or some external structures I can't cope with."

This example illustrates how partners' different conceptions of how the illness affects each other as individuals can be a source of disagreements about one partner's illness. Different ideas about time (or temporal incongruence) can promote focusing on the illness as an individual issue. Because intimates do not share similar ways of thinking about and structuring time, conflict emerges when making daily schedules and projecting timetables. Charmaz (1991) explains that the woman wants life to be the way it used to be, adhering to the old timetable when her husband was working, although he now has a time-out period for convalescing. In this case, time may never be the way it was. If they cannot discuss their differences and adopt similar frameworks with regard to the illness and how it affects their visions of the future, this will lead them to grow further apart. Further, coming to an agreement about time implies that they share similar perspectives of their future relationship. Clearly, these spouses do not view the husband's illness as a problem they will handle together.

The following example illustrates explicit and implicit talking. It is a description of spouses' use of communal coping, taken from Lyons and Meade (1995, p. 207).

> I remember going to my husband's work. I took him aside and asked him to come into the cafeteria with me. And I said, "I have MS." And I still remember, he hugged me and he said, "We'll deal with this together" and boy, did that mean a lot!

Here the husband talks explicitly about the relationship by stating what they will do together. He also talks implicitly about the relationship by using *we* as the subject instead of *you* or *I*. This relationship is not threatened by the stress of chronic illness. It is obvious that these two couples are on two different trajectories. Is it possible that their coping was incongruent (Revenson, 1994) before one partner became ill and that the stress of the illness is exaggerating or exacerbating the closeness (or distance) they had before the illness? The research designed to answer such a question is equivocal. Some studies show that couples who do well in the face of chronic illness were doing well before the diagnosis (Coyne & Fiske, 1992; Stern & Pascale, 1979; Wellisch, Jamison, & Pasnau, 1978), whereas others find that couples who were doing poorly before the diagnosis are better adjusted after the diagnosis than couples who were initially doing well (Litman, 1979; Schmaling & Sher, 2000). Although we have no idea how the couples functioned before diagnosis, by observing their conversations in these examples, we can surmise how their relationships are faring after the diagnosis. The first couple, who took an individual focus toward illness, seemed to be doing poorly in the relationship, whereas the second couple, who took a relationship approach, seemed to be doing very well.

When thinking leads to talking about the relationship, and in the case of illness, the disease's implications for the relationship, such talking can lead to better outcomes for the relationship. In the example described above in which the husband takes a relationship approach, he talks explicitly and implicitly about the relationship. However, we could presume he was thinking in implicit terms, which led him to his supposedly rapid response in relationship terms ("We'll deal with this together"). So by keeping the relationship in implicit awareness, he may have been primed to talk in relationship terms. In studies of healthy couples, talking and thinking positively about the relationship leads to better relationship outcomes (Acitelli et al., 1999; Cate et al., 1995), especially when the partners are high in *couple identity* or a sense of *we-ness*. The couple in the second example might exemplify how keeping a couple's identity in implicit awareness leads to problem solving.

What happens when explicit thinking does not lead to talking? We propose that such a situation could be detrimental to the relationship, especially in a stressful situation such as dealing with a chronic illness. If one partner keeps thoughts about the relationship from the other in times of stress, the couple misses an opportunity to discuss or resolve a relationship issue together. Next we provide an example of thinking explicitly about the relationship but not talking about it. This example also illustrates that relationship talk is not always positive. In this example, also taken from Charmaz (1991, p. 81), the husband has a spinal cord tumor that has caused paralysis of his arms and legs.

> During the course of the day, I usually ask Yolanda [his wife] for dozens of small services, over and above the main care she gives me. Since I know she

is overburdened, I generally hesitate to ask for things and feel slightly guilty about bothering her—a guilt that becomes added to that caused by my damaged body. As a result, I am especially sensitive to the tone of her response. Do I detect a note of impatience? Is she annoyed? Is she over-tired? Should I have asked her? Does that slight inflection say, "What the hell does he want from me now?"

This is an example of explicit thinking about the relationship in which the husband is thinking about how his wife is reacting to him but does not ask her how she feels. She may feel angry but does not want to upset him. He senses her anger and seems afraid to ask. His explicit thinking does not lead to explicit talking. This lack of verbal communication will presumably lead to creating more distance between husband and wife.

The final example of implicit thinking about the relationship is also taken from the work of Charmaz (1991, p. 144). The woman (Patricia) has multiple sclerosis.

> Including others in a task simplifies it and simultaneously maintains the social relationship. Patricia said, "With David's [her husband] schedule, I don't plan things like real elaborate meals during the week because I never know when he's going to leave the office. So rather than putting an additional stress on me, I don't start to cook until he comes home. We cook together; it is a good time for us, you know, we can talk, catch up on what's happened during the day. It's a real good time and I wonder why we didn't do this all along."

Although this is explicit talk about the relationship to the interviewer, the description of the activity takes a more implicit stance toward the relationship. What Patricia and David do together as a couple is "a real good time," not talking about the relationship. Thus, in cases such as this, implicit thinking about the relationship without talking about it can lead to positive outcomes for the relationship.

Relationship Awareness and Gender

Previous research has found that women in North American cultures focus more attention on relationships than men do (Acitelli, 1992; Burnett, 1987; Cate et al., 1995) and engage more in thinking positively about their relationships than men do (Cate et al., 1995). Research has shown that women tend to be the nurturers in relationships even when they are ill (Revenson, 1994, 2003, chap. 7, this volume). In Lyons et al. (1995), one woman was so concerned about the way her friends and family would react to her diagnosis of multiple sclerosis, she devised a way to disclose it to them to cause the least discomfort for them. She telephoned everyone close to her and told them about her diagnosis. Then she asked them to call her back in two weeks, which would give them time to digest the news and keep them from feeling obligated to say something immediately. In other words, she was taking care of her friends even when she was ill.

Although several research studies indicate that women think and talk about relationships more than men do, what is more interesting is that such thinking and talking seems to affect men and women differently and that talking about one's relationship is viewed in different ways by men and women. Women view relationship talk as part of everyday relationship maintenance, whereas men value it to the extent that it is used strategically to solve a relationship problem. This difference suggests a particular view that is necessary to engage both partners in coping with the illness. If both partners see the illness as a problem for the relationship, rather than just a problem for one individual, they are both more likely to realize the need to engage in relationship talk as a form of strategic relationship maintenance.

However, the literature goes beyond gender differences in thinking about relationships to suggest differences in orientations toward relationships (Peplau & Gordon, 1985). That is, it is important not only to look at differences between men and women but also differences between men and women in the ways that relationship-oriented behaviors, perceptions, and thoughts are associated with relationship satisfaction. For example, a study of perceptions of conflict (Acitelli, Douvan, & Veroff, 1993) showed that husbands' marital satisfaction was best predicted by husbands' and wives' separate reports of their own behaviors during conflict. In contrast, wives' marital satisfaction was best predicted by the *congruence* of the spouses' reports. That is, wives' understanding of their husbands (i.e., her reports of his behavior match his reports of his own behavior), perceived similarity, and actual similarity were more important to wives' satisfaction, whereas the separate, individual reports of conflict behaviors were more predictive of husbands' marital satisfaction. The finding that wives' understanding was more predictive of marital satisfaction could indicate a power differential in the relationship. The importance of understanding might indicate the need to be empowered in a marriage in which traditionally the husband has more power.

An earlier study on relationship awareness found that the extent to which husbands talked about the relationship (in an open-ended interview) was associated with wives' marital happiness, although such talk from either spouse had no link to husbands' happiness (Acitelli, 1992). Similarly, studies of social support in marriage (Acitelli & Antonucci, 1994; Julien & Markman, 1991) have demonstrated that spousal supportiveness contributes more to a woman's marital satisfaction than it does to a man's.

Taking a more cognitive perspective, Scott, Fuhrman, and Wyer (1991) have shown that women are more likely than men to store conversations with partners as relationship memories, whereas men are more likely to store them in terms of the issue discussed. Presumably, then, there are more situations for women that trigger thoughts about the relationship. Perhaps the more interactions that have implications for the relationship, the higher the probability that perceived interactions with a spouse can influence one's satisfaction with the relationship. For example, when a husband provides comfort to his wife when she is ill, his providing comfort may stimulate different thoughts in each partner. The husband may think it is unfortunate that his wife is ill, and the wife may think that she is pleased her husband is showing that he cares about her. Whereas the wife may see her illness as a challenge for the relationship, the husband may view the illness as a problem without relationship implications. Acitelli and Antonucci (1994) speculated that men may not make as strong a connection between perceived support and relationship satisfaction as women do. As social support is more salient to women than men (Sarason, Sarason, & Pierce, 1994), it is reasonable to suggest that social support in marriage would affect women's more than men's satisfaction with relationships. Likewise, in a study of young married couples, Acitelli (1992) found that the more the husband attended to the marital relationship, the happier the wife was with regard to both her marriage and her life.

Levenson, Carstensen, and Gottman (1993) come to a similar conclusion: Wives' physical and psychological health are more closely tied to marital satisfaction than are husbands'. They explain that when a marriage is in trouble, wives take on the emotional work of repairing it, whereas husbands are more likely to withdraw. This withdrawal not only buffers husbands from the unhealthy consequences but adds to the wives' emotional burden as well. Thus, when marriages are distressed, wives' health suffers (see also Gove, Hughes, & Style, 1983; Kessler, 1991).

An Investigation of Health, Gender, and Relationship Talk

In this section we present data from an empirical investigation that addresses the relationship between gender and relationship talk. The study compares married couples in which one spouse is chronically ill with a sample of healthy couples. Using these data we examine general coping styles of husbands and wives with a special emphasis on which spouse is ill, as well as the *explicit talk* form of relationship awareness.

The study that we report (Badr, 2002) focuses on the challenges that marriages face when one spouse has a chronic illness. Specifically, which spouse is sick makes a difference in relationship outcomes because of the traditional roles men and women are accustomed to playing. Studies have shown differences between men and women with regard to coping and support processes in relationships (Bem, 1993; Gore & Colton, 1991; Gottlieb & Wagner, 1991; Gottman, 1991; Vaux, 1985). Moreover, the associations between marital quality and health appear to be stronger for women than for men (Burman & Margolin, 1992; Kiecolt-Glaser & Newton, 2001). In chronic illness, Hagedoorn, Buunk, Kuijer, Wobbes, and Sanderman (2000) demonstrated that both female patients and female partners of patients perceive more psychological distress and a lower quality of life than women in healthy couples.

Data were collected data from 182 married couples. Of these, 90 couples were categorized as healthy couples (in which both spouses were healthy), and 92 couples were classified as chronic illness couples because one spouse (50 wives, 42 husbands) had a chronic illness. A wide range of chronic illnesses were represented, with one fourth of the sample having cancer. Both members of the couple were asked to complete a confidential survey.

Gender Differences in Styles of Coping With Illness

According to Lyons and Sullivan (1998), three approaches have been used to study psychosocial adaptation to chronic illness. The individual perspective focuses on assessment of illness related stressors and helping patients, spouses, and their loved ones cope with illness or disability in their lives (e.g.,

Thompson, 1996). The social change perspective is concerned with the social construction of illness, focusing on the need to change societal values, social policies, and social services for the ill and disabled (e.g., Duval, 1984; Wolfensberger, 1983). The relationship perspective proposes that chronic illness or disability is an interpersonal issue rather than an individual issue. The quality of relationships thus plays an important role in helping individuals and families cope with, adapt to, and perhaps even survive chronic illness (e.g., Atkins, Kaplan, & Toshima, 1991; Coyne et al., 2001; Lyons, Mickelson, Sullivan, & Coyne, 1998; Manne, Alfieri, Taylor, & Dougherty, 1999).

Assessing coping within the context of relationships poses a challenge for researchers because the lines separating *what is good for me* from *what is good for my spouse or good for the relationship* become easily blurred. For example, husbands who protectively buffer their wives by not telling them about a bad test result may, on the one hand, be engaging in relationship-focused coping because they do not want to upset their wives (Coyne & Smith, 1991, 1994). At the same time, not telling their wives may help husbands to escape the problem by not addressing it, which could be indicative of emotion-focused escape–avoidance coping. In this way, coping behaviors might actually serve dual functions in romantic relationships (for a similar argument, see Pierce, Sarason, & Sarason, 1991).

Currently, no single instrument exists that simultaneously assesses problem-, emotion-, and relationship-focused coping. A cursory examination of existing measures indicates some degree of overlap in items classified as different types of coping behaviors. For example, it is equally plausible to assume that a person would consider the item "deny or hide my worries," a protective-buffering statement taken from the Relationship-Focused Coping Scale (Coyne & Smith, 1991), as meaning the same thing as "I've been refusing to believe that it has happened," an emotion-focused coping item from the Brief COPE (Carver, 1997). Having a single instrument that assesses different types of coping might help not only to determine and perhaps eliminate some of this overlap but also to clarify our understanding of coping process within the marital context.

Despite the fact that the majority of research emerging from the relationship perspective focuses on social support processes, we still know very little about how couples can effectively maintain their relationship while trying to manage a chronic illness (Heller & Rook, 1997; Vaux, 1988). Although many different factors can potentially influence this process, one factor may be the gender of the ill spouse. For the most part, researchers who examine gender and coping have not examined husbands and wives in both the patient and the well-spouse role within the same study (see Revenson, 1994, chap. 7, this volume, for a discussion of this issue). As such, it becomes difficult to tease apart gender from other potential variables such as health status in understanding how couples cope. Despite this, studies that have examined husbands' or wives' coping separately seem to suggest that husbands' engage in problem-focused coping whether or not they are ill, whereas wives' coping may change depending on the demands of the illness situation (e.g., Coyne & Smith, 1991, 1994; Lichtman, Taylor, & Wood, 1987). More studies are needed that include both healthy and chronic illness couples with husbands and wives in both the well-spouse and the patient role in order to determine whether this is the case.

To this end, the goals of Badr's (2002) study were threefold. First, she combined existing coping measures to reduce overlap among items and take into account the relational context and its role in the coping process. Second, she investigated whether husbands and wives exhibit different orientations to coping depending on whether they are healthy or ill. Third, she attempted to discover whether different coping styles are related to marital adjustment using both members of the dyad and comparing couples in which the husband is ill with couples in which the wife is ill.

An abridged measure that simultaneously taps emotion-, problem-, and relationship-focused coping was created from factor analysis of the items on Carver's (1997) Brief COPE and Coyne and Smith's (1991) Relationship-Focused Coping Scale. Coping styles were divided into two types: Intrapersonal Coping (individual or solitary coping) and Interpersonal Coping (communication between partners, including the strategies of active engagement, approach coping, and seeking social support). Interpersonal coping was significantly positively associated and intrapersonal coping was significantly negatively associated with marital satisfaction for both husbands and wives.

A series of repeated measures analyses revealed that ill wives were less likely than ill husbands to use interpersonal coping as a strategy, whereas well wives were more likely than well husbands to employ these same strategies. Active engagement was associated with marital satisfaction among chronic illness couples but not healthy couples. Specifically, wives' use of active engagement as a form of coping was associated with greater marital satisfaction for both husbands and wives when the wife was ill and greater marital satisfaction for husbands when the husband was ill. These analyses suggest that couples were more satisfied when they employed coping strategies that involved actively confronting problems and openly expressing feelings. At the same time, couples were less satisfied when they employed intrapersonal coping strategies that were more solitary in nature, such as avoidance coping, and interpersonal coping strategies that involved masking feelings and protective buffering, especially when the wife was ill.

Gender and Relationship Talk in the Illness Context

We also examined the role of relationship talk when one spouse has a chronic illness. Maintaining spousal communication becomes especially critical in the face of chronic illness because opportunities for couples to interact physically or to spend time together engaging in leisure activities may become limited because of the illness.

When couples talk together in relational terms, that is, when they talk about themselves as a couple or about the relationship as an entity, it indicates attention to the relationship (Acitelli, 1992; Acitelli & Badr, 2000). Relationship talk focuses solely on the relationship and is important because the consequences of such talk are different than when the focus is on individual partners. For example, couples in conflict are less likely to remain in conflict if the focus of their conversations can shift from an individual partner (partner blame) to the relationship (Acitelli, 1988, 1992; Bernal & Baker, 1979). A general expectation is that the more couples talk together about their relationship in the face of chronic illness, the better their marital adjustment. Engaging in relationship talk might buffer couples from the negative consequences of chronic illness on their marriages as well as on their mental health.

Again, we expected the gender of the ill spouse to influence our findings. For example, a study of glioma patients and their spouses showed that when wives were the patients, they were eight times more likely to be separated or divorced than when husbands were the patients (Cross et al., 2001). This finding could be interpreted to mean that couples may be more likely to experience distress when wives rather than husbands are ill. Other studies have found greater problems with adjustment (Siegel, Karus, Raveis, Christ, & Mesagno, 1996) and caregiver burden (Gilbar, 1999) in well husbands.

We first examined whether wives' engagement in relationship talk buffered them from the negative association between physical health and mental health. Relationship talk was measured using five items regarding the frequency of relationship talk taken from the Acitelli (1997) Couples and Well-Being Project and The Early Years of Marriage Project (Veroff, Douvan, & Hatchett, 1995). Participants were asked to rate on a Likert-type scale, the frequency with which they engaged in various types of relationship talk with their spouse. Consistent with the literature, we found that for healthy wives, the more they engaged their ill husbands in relationship talk, the better their mental health. However, this finding did not hold for the ill wives whose mental health was poorer.

We next examined whether husbands' engagement in relationship talk buffered them from the negative effects of illness on mental health. Results indicated that husbands' engagement in relationship talk had little effect on the mental health of husbands in healthy couples or husbands whose wives were chronically ill. However, the more ill husbands talked, the better was their mental health.

We also conducted analyses to determine whether engagement in relationship talk would buffer husbands and wives from the negative effects of illness on relationship satisfaction. Wives' engagement in relationship talk had a main effect on both husbands' and wives' relationship satisfaction. Even though wives' engagement in relationship talk was related to both husbands' and wives' overall relationship satisfaction, it did not buffer either wives or husbands from feeling bad about their marital relationship if they were the chronically ill partner.

The more husbands engaged in relationship talk, the happier they were in their marriages. Well husbands were happiest overall when they engaged in more relationship talk, and well husbands who talked least were the unhappiest. Similarly, the more husbands engaged in relationship talk, the more satisfied their wives were in the relationship. Ill wives were happiest when their husbands engaged in more relationship talk and were the least satisfied of all four groups when their husbands engaged in less relationship talk. Engagement in relationship talk was thus found to be the most beneficial to relationships in which the wife was ill and the husband was well.

Even though wives' talk fostered positive relationship outcomes in general, it did not buffer couples from the negative consequences of the illness on overall marital satisfaction. Husbands' talk, on the other hand, did buffer both husbands and wives from the negative consequences of illness on marital satisfaction and, in addition, buffered husbands from the negative consequences of illness on mental health. Moreover, husbands' talk seems to be particularly important for couples in which the wife was ill. This is consistent with earlier research on relationship talk in general, which shows that the happiest wives are those whose husbands talked more about the relationship than the wives themselves did (Acitelli, 1992).

When husbands are ill, their own engagement in relationship talk may assist them in communicating their support needs and help them to solve problems before they become a threat to the relationship. This is beneficial to their own mental health, their wives' mental health, and the overall quality of the marital relationship. When wives are ill, husbands' engagement in relationship talk may help both partners to better understand one another's behaviors and responses to the illness situation. When husbands step outside their gendered roles in relationships and take on some of the responsibilities of maintaining the relationship when their wives are unable to because of their illness, their wives are more likely to respond positively. Moreover, husbands who take a more active role in maintaining the relationship may feel a renewed sense of commitment and love toward their partners.

Summary

How couples cope with chronic illness may depend, to some extent, on who is the well spouse and who is the ill spouse. We addressed the need for investigating the idea that men and women behave differently and expect different things from their partners depending on whether they are in the role of the patient or the well spouse.

In general, if partners talk about the relationship, the less likely their health will influence their marital satisfaction. More specifically, the more husbands engaged in relationship talk, the happier the marriage, especially for ill wives. Women, with their interdependent approach to relationships, are likely to see such attention, if they get it, as having good implications for their relationship, whereas ill men may focus more on whether such attention makes them feel better about life in general. Yet if ill spouses, regardless of gender, have greater emotional needs and their well spouses take a more traditional gender role approach to relationships, women are likely to suffer more than men when they are ill. Men may have good intentions by using such coping strategies as engaging in problem solving or sharing activities, thinking perhaps that they are protecting their partners by not talking about feelings or the relationship. Women, on the other hand, may interpret such behaviors as ignoring their feelings, and consequently, such behaviors may have negative implications for the marital relationship. Women in the well-spouse role, however, were more likely to cope by giving emotional support through talking.

The more husbands discuss their relationships with their wives during times of stress (chronic illness), the less likely a mismatch of support will occur, paving the way for positive relationship outcomes. This is true regardless of whether the husband or wife is ill. Our data provide evidence that chronic illness needs to be seen not only as an individual challenge but a relationship challenge as well.

Although our research addressed only one form of relationship awareness (explicit talking), the other forms of relationship awareness, explicit thinking, implicit thinking, and talking, also suggest directions for future research. If a person thinks explicitly about the relationship without talking about it, it could signify a lack of communication that leads to more distance between partners. If either partner ruminates about how the illness has interfered with their relationship and does not share these feeling, the fears and emotions can incubate and make the problem even larger than it really is. However, as we have seen here, talking explicitly about the relationship can lead to positive outcomes in both relationship satisfaction and individual well-being. Other research on implicit thinking and talking about the relationship (Acitelli et al., 1999) suggests that taking an implicit relationship stance, seeing problems as our problems, whether thinking or talking, can lead to positive outcomes. Although conflicts are inevitable, if both partners see the illness as *our* illness, the illness routines become shared. Rather than two individuals going their separate ways, the spouses are more likely see themselves as a team, solving problems together.

References

Acitelli, L. K. (1988). When spouses talk to each other about their relationship. *Journal of Social and Personal Relationships, 5*, 185–199.

Acitelli, L. K. (1992). Gender differences in relationship awareness and marital satisfaction among young married couples. *Personality & Social Psychology Bulletin, 18*, 102–110.

Acitelli, L. K. (1997). Sampling couples to understand them: Mixing the theoretical with the practical. *Journal of Social and Personal Relationships, 14*, 243–261.

Acitelli, L. K., & Antonucci, T. C. (1994). Gender differences in the link between marital support and satisfaction in older couples. *Journal of Personality and Social Psychology, 67*, 688–698.

Acitelli, L. K., & Badr, H. (2000, September). *Perspectives on relationship awareness and satisfaction: Implications for coping.* Paper presented at the International Workshop on Stress and Coping in Couples, University of Fribourg, Fribourg, Switzerland.

Acitelli, L. K., Douvan, E., & Veroff, J. (1993). Perception of self and spouse during conflict: How important are similarity and understanding? *Journal of Social & Personal Relationships, 10*, 1–14.

Acitelli, L. K., Rogers, S., & Knee, C. R. (1999). The role of relational identity in the link between relationship thinking and relationship satisfaction. *Journal of Social & Personal Relationships, 16*, 591–618.

Atkins, C. J., Kaplan, R. M., & Toshima, M. T. (1991). Close relationships in the epidemiology of cardiovascular disease. In W. H. Jones & D. Perlman (Eds.), *Advances in personal relationships* (Vol. 3, pp. 207–231). London: Kingsley.

Badr, H. (2002). *Chronic illness as a relationship challenge.* Unpublished doctoral dissertation, University of Houston, Houston, TX.

Bem, S. L. (1993). *The lenses of gender: Transforming the debate on sexual inequality.* New Haven, CT: Yale University Press.

Bernal, G., & Baker, J. (1979). Toward a metacommunicational framework of couple interaction. *Family Process, 18*, 293–302.

Burnett, R. (1987). Reflection in personal relationships. In R. Burnett, P. McGhee, & D. C. Clarke (Eds.), *Accounting for relationships: Explanation, representation and knowledge*. London: Methuen.

Burman, B., & Margolin, G. (1992). Analysis of the association between marital relationships and health problems: An interactional perspective. *Psychological Bulletin, 112*, 39–63.

Carver, C. S. (1997). You want to measure coping but your protocol's too long: Consider the Brief COPE. *International Journal of Behavioral Medicine, 4*, 92–100.

Cate, R. M., Koval, J. E., Lloyd, S. A., & Wilson, G. (1995). The assessment of relationship thinking in dating relationships. *Personal Relationships, 2*, 77–95.

Charmaz, K. (1991). *Good days, bad days: The self in chronic illness and time*. New Brunswick, NJ: Rutgers University Press.

Coyne, J. C., & Fiske, V. (1992). Couples coping with chronic and catastrophic illness. In T. J. Akamatsu, M. A. P. Stephens, S. E. Hobfoll, & J. H. Crowther (Eds.), *Family health psychology* (pp. 129–149). Washington, DC: Hemisphere Publication Services.

Coyne, J. C., Rohrbaugh, M. J., Shoham, V., Sonnega, J. S., Nicklas, J. M., & Cranford, J. A. (2001). Prognostic importance of marital quality for survival of congestive heart failure. *The American Journal of Cardiology, 88*, 526–529.

Coyne, J. C., & Smith, D. A. F. (1991). Couples coping with a myocardial infarction: A contextual perspective on wives' distress. *Journal of Personality and Social Psychology, 61*, 404–412.

Coyne, J. C., & Smith, D. A. F. (1994). Couples coping with myocardial infarction: Contextual perspective on patient self-efficacy. *Journal of Family Psychology, 8*, 1–13.

Cross, N., Glantz, M., Cole, B., Cobb, J., Recht, L., Edwards, K., & Chamberlain, M. (2001). Dramatically increased frequency of divorce and separation in female but not male patients with gliomas. *Neurology, 56*, A477.

Dainton, M., & Stafford, L. (1993). Routine maintenance behaviors: A comparison of relationship type, partner similarity and sex differences. *Journal of Social and Personal Relationships, 10*, 255–271.

Duval, M. L. (1984). Psychosocial metaphors of physical distress among MS patients. *Social Science and Medicine, 19*, 635–638.

Frisbie, W. P., Optiz, W., & Kelly, W. R. (1985). Marital instability trends among Mexican Americans as compared to Blacks and Anglos: New evidence. *Social Science Quarterly, 66*, 587–601.

Gilbar, O. (1999). Gender as a predictor of burden and psychological distress of elderly husbands and wives of cancer patients. *Psycho-Oncology, 8*, 287–294.

Gore, S., & Colton, M. E. (1991). Gender, stress and distress: Social-relational influences. In J. Eckenrode (Ed.), *The social context of coping* (pp. 139–163). New York: Plenum Press.

Gottlieb, B. H., & Wagner, F. (1991). Stress and support processes in close relationships. In J. Eckenrode (Ed.), *The social context of coping* (pp. 165–188). New York: Plenum Press.

Gottman, J. M. (1991). Predicting the longitudinal course of marriages. *Journal of Marital and Family Therapy, 17*, 3–7.

Gove, W. R., Hughes, M., & Style, C. B. (1983). Does marriage have positive effects on the psychological well-being of the individual? *Journal of Health and Social Behavior, 24*, 122–131.

Hagedoorn, M., Buunk, B. P., Kuijer, R. G., Wobbes, T., & Sanderman, R. (2000). Couples dealing with cancer: Role and gender differences regarding psychological distress and quality of life. *Psycho-Oncology, 9*, 232–242.

Heller, K., & Rook, K. S. (1997). Distinguishing the theoretive functions of social ties. In S. Duck (Ed.), *Handbook of personal relationships* (2nd ed., pp. 648–670). Chichester, England: Wiley.

Julien, D., & Markman, H. J. (1991). Social support and social networks as determinants of individual and marital outcomes. *Journal of Social and Personal Relationships, 8*, 548–568.

Kayser, K., Sormanti, M., & Strainchamps, E. (1999). Women coping with cancer: The influence of relationship factors on psychosocial adjustment. *Psychology of Women Quarterly, 23*, 725–739.

Kessler, R. C. (1991). Perceived support and adjustment to stress: Methodological considerations. In H.O.F. Vieil & U. Baumann (Eds.), *The meaning and measurement of social support* (pp. 259–271). New York: Hemisphere Publication Services.

Kiecolt-Glaser, J. K., & Newton, T. L. (2001). Marriage and health: His and hers. *Psychological Bulletin, 127*, 472–503.

Levenson, R. W., Carstensen, L. L., & Gottman, J. M. (1993). Long-term marriage: Age, gender, and satisfaction. *Psychology and Aging, 8,* 301–313.

Lichtman, R. R., Taylor, S. E., & Wood, J. V. (1987). Social support and marital adjustment after breast cancer. *Journal of Psychosocial Oncology, 5,* 47–74.

Litman, T. J. (1979). The family in health and health care: A socio-behavioral overview. In E. G. Jaco (Ed.), *Patients, physicians, and illness* (pp. 69–101). New York: Free Press.

Lyons, R., & Meade, D. (1995). Painting a new face on relationships: Relationship remodeling in response to chronic illness. In S. Duck & J. T. Wood (Eds.), *Confronting relationship challenges.* Thousand Oaks, CA: Sage.

Lyons, R., Mickelson, K. D., Sullivan, M. J. L., & Coyne, J. C. (1998). Coping as a communal process. *Journal of Social & Personal Relationships, 15,* 579–605.

Lyons, R., & Sullivan, M. J. L. (1998). Curbing loss in illness and disability: A relationship perspective. In J. H. Harvey (Ed.), *Perspectives on personal and interpersonal loss: A sourcebook* (pp. 137–152). Bristol, PA: Taylor & Francis.

Lyons, R., Sullivan, M. J. L., Ritvo, P., & Coyne, J. C. (Eds.). (1995). *Relationships in chronic illness and disability.* Thousand Oaks, CA: Sage.

Manne, S. L., Alfieri, T., Taylor, K. L., & Dougherty, J. (1999). Spousal negative responses to cancer patients: The role of social restriction, spouse mood, and relationship satisfaction. *Journal of Consulting and Clinical Psychology, 67,* 352–361.

Peplau, L. A., & Gordon, S. L. (1985). Women and men in love: Sex differences in close heterosexual relationships. In V. E. O'Leary, R. K. Unger, & B. S. Wallston (Eds.), *Women, gender and social psychology* (pp. 257–292). Hillsdale, NJ: Erlbaum.

Pierce, G. R., Sarason, B. R., & Sarason, I. G. (1991). General and relationship-based perceptions of social support: Are two constructs better than one? *Journal of Personality and Social Psychology, 61,* 1028–1039.

Polanyi, M. (1966). *The tacit dimension.* Garden City, NY: Doubleday.

Revenson, T. A. (1994). Social support and marital coping with chronic illness. *Annals of Behavioral Medicine, 16,* 122–130.

Revenson, T. A. (2003). Scenes from a marriage: Examining support, coping, and gender within the context of chronic illness. In J. Suls & K. Wallston (Eds.), *Social psychological foundations of health and illness* (pp. 530–559). Oxford, England: Blackwell Publishing.

Sabogal, F., Marin, G., Otero-Sabogal, R., Marin, B. V., & Perez-Stable, E. J. (1987). Hispanic familism and acculturation: What changes and what doesn't? *Hispanic Journal of Behavioral Sciences, 9,* 397–412.

Sarason, I. G., Sarason, B. R., & Pierce, G. R. (1994). Social support: Global and relationship-based levels of analysis. *Journal of Social and Personal Relationships, 11,* 295–312.

Schmaling, K. B., & Sher, T. G. (2000). *The psychology of couples and illness.* Washington, DC: American Psychological Association.

Scott, C. K., Fuhrman, R. W., & Wyer, R. S. (1991). Information processing in close relationships. In G. J. O. Fletcher & F. D. Fincham (Eds.), *Cognition in close relationships* (pp. 36–67). Hillsdale, NJ: Erlbaum.

Siegel, K., Karus, D. G., Raveis, V. H., Christ, G. H., & Mesagno, F. P. (1996). Depressive distress among the spouses of terminally ill cancer patients. *Cancer Practice, 4*(1), 25–30.

Stern, M. J., & Pascale, L. (1979). Psychosocial adaptation to post-myocardial infarction: The spouse's dilemma. *Journal of Psychosomatic Research, 23,* 83–87.

Thompson, S. C. (1996). Barriers to maintaining a sense of meaning and control in the face of loss. *Journal of Personal and Interpersonal Loss, 1,* 333–357.

Vaux, A. (1985). Variations in social support associated with gender, ethnicity, and age. *Journal of Social Issues, 41,* 89–110.

Vaux, A. (1988). *Social support: Theory, research and intervention.* New York: Praeger Publishers.

Veroff, J., Douvan, L., & Hatchett, S. J. (1995). *Marital instability: The early years.* New York: Praeger Publishers.

Wegner, D. M., & Giuliano, T. (1982). The forms of social awareness. In W. J. Ickes (Ed.), *Personality, roles, and social behavior* (pp. 165–198). New York: Springer-Verlag.

Wellisch, D. K., Jamison, R., & Pasnau, R. O. (1978). Psychosocial aspects of mastectomy II: The man's perspective. *American Journal of Psychiatry, 135,* 543–545.

Wolfensberger, W. (1983). Social role valorization: A proposed new term for the principle of normalization. *Mental Retardation, 21,* 235–239.

7

Couples Coping With Chronic Illness: What's Gender Got to Do With It?

*Tracey A. Revenson, Ana F. Abraído-Lanza,
S. Deborah Majerovitz, and Caren Jordan*

Over the past decade, the lion's share of research on coping has focused on individual coping efforts and adaptation outcomes. However, major life stressors are not experienced in a social vacuum. When one family member is experiencing ongoing, complex stressors or life strains, other family members are affected by both the stressor itself, its psychological impact on the affected individual, and its effect on the family's functioning. At this juncture in *stress and coping* research, it is important to move past a dominant focus on individual-level processes into a social ecological or family systems framework.

Marriage is a primary relationship often considered distinct from other family relationships because it is long-term, affords a central role identity, and provides a fundamental resource of social support and coping assistance (Revenson, 1994). Much research has demonstrated the beneficial effects of social support from family on patients' coping, across a number of chronic conditions (e.g., Cutrona, 1996; Lyons, Sullivan, Ritvo, & Coyne, 1996; Revenson, 2003). Far less research has focused on the effect of illness on the healthy spouse, children, the marriage, or the family (Pedersen & Revenson, in press).

Husbands and wives experience unique stresses as a result of living with a chronically ill person (see chap. 6, this volume; Hagedoorn, Kuijer, Buunk, DeJong, Wobbes, & Sanderman, 2000; Revenson & Gibofsky, 1995; Revenson & Majerovitz, 1990, 1991). Some stresses emanate directly from caregiving in which spouses are inextricably involved in decision making about treatment and day-to-day care if the patient is disabled. Other stresses emerge from the need to restructure family roles and responsibilities as the disease progresses

The original research described in this chapter was funded by grants from the Cornell University Medical College Arthritis and Musculoskeletal Disease Center (AR38520), the City University of New York PSC-CUNY Research Award Program, and the New York Chapter of the Arthritis Foundation to Tracey A. Revenson, as well as summer student grants from the New York Chapter of the Arthritis Foundation to Ana F. Abraído-Lanza, S. Deborah Majerovitz, and Caren Jordan. We would also like to acknowledge Chandra Mason, Judith Schor, and Vita Rabinowitz for their intellectual and analytical contributions to the couples study. We thank Allan Gibofsky and Stephen Paget of the Hospital for Special Surgery in New York City for assistance and sage guidance during the entire project.

or presents new challenges. Still other stresses are filtered through the lens of the patient's experience, as in the case of a healthy spouse feeling helpless at seeing her or his partner in pain. There are also societal or normative expectations that spouses care for their ill partner. In fact, the provision of support may be conceptualized as a stressor for the spouse in its own right, particularly when, as in the case of chronic illness, it is a lifelong task.

Spouses and others in committed relationships, such as domestic partnerships, are faced with dual challenges in the coping process: as the primary provider of support to the ill partner and as a family member who needs support in coping with the illness-related stresses she or he is experiencing. Individual coping choices not only affect both partners' health and well-being but also affect the marital relationship (see chap. 2, this volume).

In this chapter, we address several issues in the conceptualization and study of dyadic coping with specific illustrations from the literature on couples coping with illness. First we describe several nascent theoretical approaches to dyadic coping. We then explore the "missing" variable of gender from research on couples who are coping with illness by examining coping from two perspectives that are extremely gendered—one that has been studied before, social support, and one that has not been found under the rubric of coping, division of labor. We end with a blueprint for future research on couples' coping that incorporates gender.

Conceptual Models of Marital Coping

In the past decade, a number of studies have examined couples coping with illness at the dyadic level of analysis. This research has studied heart disease (Coyne et al., 2001; Coyne & Smith, 1991, 1994; Lyons, Mickelson, Sullivan, & Coyne, 1998; Michela, 1987; Rankin-Esquer, Deeter, & Taylor, 2000; Rohrbaugh et al., 2002; Rose, Suls, Green, Lounsbury, & Gordon, 1996; Suls, Green, Rose, Lounsbury, & Gordon, 1997), end-stage renal disease (Gray, Brogan, & Kutner, 1985), infertility (Berghuis & Stanton, 2002; Levin, Sher, & Theodos, 1997; Pasch & Christensen, 2000); rheumatoid arthritis (Bermas, Tucker, Winkelman, & Katz, 2000; Danoff-Burg & Revenson, 2000; Manne & Zautra, 1989, 1990; Revenson, 1994, 2003; Tucker, Winkelman, Katz, & Bermas, 1999) and cancer (Baider, Koch, Eascson, & Kaplan De-Nour, 1998; Baider, Perez, & Kaplan De-Nour, 1989; Hagedoorn, Kuijer, et al., 2000; Halford, Scott, & Smythe, 2000; Manne, Alfieri, Taylor, & Dougherty, 1999; Manne & Glassman, 2000; Northouse, Templin, & Mood, 2001; Northouse, Templin, Mood, & Oberst, 1995; Pistrang & Barker, 1995; Zunkel, 2002), as well as other health conditions (Schmaling & Sher, 2000). These studies can be characterized by three different, though somewhat overlapping, approaches to couples' coping: relationship-focused coping, mutual influence, and coping congruence (fit). All three approaches can be applied to couples confronting a health-related stressor; all integrate elements of family systems theory; and all require data from both husbands and wives in their research endeavors.

Relationship-Focused Coping

An exciting approach to couples' coping focuses on maintaining the quality of the marital relationship as part of the coping process (see chap. 3, this volume; Coyne & Fiske, 1992; DeLongis & O'Brien, 1990; Lyons et al., 1998; O'Brien & DeLongis, 1996, 1997). This approach expands the stress and coping paradigm developed by Richard Lazarus (Lazarus, 1981, 1999; Lazarus & Folkman, 1984; Lazarus & Launier, 1978) to dyadic-level coping and also considers coping within an interpersonal context.

Lazarus' stress and coping paradigm has been the gold standard in the field for over 2 decades. In its most simplistic interpretation, coping strategies have been described as serving problem-focused and emotion-focused functions. Problem-focused coping efforts are aimed at managing or eliminating the source of stress; emotion-focused coping is directed toward managing the emotional distress that arises from stress appraisals. Supportive relationships are conceptualized primarily as available resources that can aid the individual's coping in a number of ways by providing (a) information about coping options; (b) feedback validating or criticizing the individual's coping choices; (c) instrumental assistance in carrying out the coping actions; or (d) emotional sustenance to help sustain coping efforts (e.g., Cutrona, 1996). As such, social support has been conceptualized as coping assistance (Thoits, 1986).

Relationship-focused coping involves a reformulation of the stress and coping paradigm to include a third coping function. When faced with a stressful situation, each partner may attend to the other's emotional needs in order to maintain the integrity of the relationship. Partners endeavor to manage their own distress without creating upset or problems for the other partner. Relationship-focused coping involves a balance between self and other, with the goal of maintaining the integrity of the marital relationship above either partner's needs. Modes of coping include negotiating or compromising with others, considering the other person's situation, and being empathic (DeLongis & O'Brien, 1990).

A few studies have examined relationship-focused coping among couples in which the husband had experienced a myocardial infarction (MI; Coyne & Smith, 1991, 1994; Suls et al., 1997).[1] These studies focused on a particular relationship-focused coping strategy, *protective buffering*, which involves "hiding concerns, denying worries, and yielding to the partner to avoid disagreements" (Coyne & Smith, 1991, p. 405). Although protective buffering is ostensibly used to avoid disagreements and "protect" the relationship, it appears to exact psychological costs for the person using it in terms of increased psychological distress. Thus, wives' coping efforts to shield husbands from stress in the post-MI period may contribute to their own distress (Coyne & Smith, 1991), as do husbands' efforts to protect their wives (Suls et al., 1997). Perhaps this happens because the partner using protective

---

[1]Another excellent research example of relationship-focused coping can be found in chapter 3 of this volume, in which Preece and DeLongis study relationship-focused coping with the interpersonal stresses experienced by stepfamilies.

buffering feels constrained in expressing negative emotions or worries to the other person (cf. Lepore's, 1997, idea of social constraints). However, protective buffering does not appear to harm the spouse, that is, the person being "protected" (Suls et al., 1997). Thus, relationship-focused coping may require a trade-off between protecting one's own well-being and that of her or his partner.

Mutual Influence Models

Mutual influence models do not specify a particular function of coping but focus on the effects of one partner's coping on the other partner's coping and adjustment (e.g., Manne & Zautra, 1990). A study of adjustment to infertility conducted by Berghuis and Stanton (2002) provides a nice illustration in that it attempts to untangle three possible mechanisms through which each partner's coping influences her or his own adjustment as well as the other partner's. The first mechanism is essentially an additive, or separate influence, model: Each person's adjustment is independently affected by her or his own coping *and* the partner's coping. The two other mechanisms are interaction models in which the relation between coping and adjustment is moderated by what the other person is (or is not) doing. One version of this interactional model posits that if partners use similar coping strategies then adjustment will be greater. The other interaction model suggests that one partner's use of an effective strategy might predominate, either nudging the other partner's coping in the same direction or "canceling out" the effects of the partner's less effective strategies. Although slightly different, both interaction mechanisms involve one partner's coping moderating the other partner's coping.

These models were tested in a prospective study of couples seeking treatment for infertility (Berghuis & Stanton, 2002). Husbands and wives completed measures of coping, depression, and marital satisfaction twice: prior to artificial insemination by the husband and after receiving a negative pregnancy test result. The findings supported all three models to some extent, but the evidence was strongest for the third model, primarily with regard to *coping through emotional approach*, a coping mode that involves both emotional processing and emotional expression. The relationship between wives' use of emotional approach coping and depression was a function of their husbands' use of that same strategy. If wives coped primarily through emotional approach, their husbands' use of that strategy was less influential on (the wife's) level of depression. Conversely, if husbands engaged in emotional approach coping, although the wives did *not*, the wives had relatively low depression scores. In other words, if wives used very little emotional approach coping, their husbands' emotional approach coping was more strongly related to the wives' depression level. If both members of the couple coped very little through emotional approach, wives were more depressed after the failed insemination attempt. This pattern of findings suggests a *compensatory coping* model, in which one person in the family has to use an effective coping strategy (effective, i.e., relative to the target stressor).

Coping Congruence

A third approach emphasizes the congruence or fit between marital partners' coping responses as a predictor of adaptation (Revenson, 1994). Conceptualizing couples' coping in terms of congruence is drawn from person–environment fit theory (French, Rodgers, & Cobb, 1974) and family systems theories (e.g., Patterson & Garwick, 1994). Within family systems theories, stressors such as illness are seen as exerting a disorganizing influence on the family, which then requires a reorganization effort, a form of coping. Thus, the goal of couples' coping is to maximize the congruence or *fit* between the partners' coping styles in order to cope most effectively *as a couple*. Strategies that work in direct opposition or cancel each other out are incongruent and would lead to worse psychosocial outcomes.

Congruence, however, can involve either similarity or complementarity of coping styles. If spouses use similar coping strategies, it might be easier to contend with stress: Coping efforts are coordinated and mutually reinforcing—that is, one partner's efforts do not impede the other's efforts. At the same time, complementary coping styles can be congruent when they work in concert to reach a desired goal, either enhancing the other person's strategy or filling a coping "gap." In fact, complementary strategies may be more effective than when husband and wife use identical strategies because the couple, as a unit, will have a broader coping repertoire. Dissimilar strategies would be seen as noncongruent if one partner's coping efforts were undermined by the other's coping efforts.

An Empirical Investigation of the Coping Congruence Model

In this investigation, we used the congruence approach to study marital coping among 113 middle-aged and older married couples who were coping with one partner's rheumatic disease (the wife in three quarters of the couples, the husband in the remaining one quarter). We refer to the person with rheumatic disease as the *patient* and the partner without rheumatic disease as *the spouse*. The measures, all self-report multi-item scales with good reliability and validity, included coping (Revised Ways of Coping Scale; WOC-revised; Folkman, Lazarus, Dunkel-Schetter, DeLongis, & Gruen, 1986), depressive symptoms (Center for Epidemiological Studies Depression Scale; CES-D; Radloff, 1977), marital functioning (Dyadic Adjustment Scale; DAS; Spanier, 1976), and mental health (Mental Health Inventory; MHI; Veit & Ware, 1983). Patients and their spouses completed all measures independently, and data were linked *within* the couple for statistical analyses, yielding a couple-level analysis.

The primary measure of coping was the Revised Ways of Coping Scale (Folkman et al., 1986), a 66-item self-report measure that contains a broad range of cognitive and behavioral strategies. We made the scale situation specific by eliciting coping responses in response to *your illness* (for the patient) or *your partner's illness* (for the spouse). Although most studies have adopted the factor structures found with samples of healthy, young-adult married couples and older couples (Folkman et al., 1986), we found these structures did not fit our data. Our own factor analysis produced a seven-factor solution that included a broad range of strategies.[2] We used cluster analysis (Aldenderfer & Blashfeld, 1984) to analyze and describe how husbands and wives coped *as a unit* with rheumatic disease. The statistical procedures leading to the final four-cluster solution are described in Revenson (2003). On the whole, the use of a single strategy or set of strategies did not characterize couples' coping profiles; instead, individuals in all four profiles used a wide range of strategies, suggesting flexible coping.

The first cluster, composed of 14 couples, was characterized as *effortful partnerships*, because of the fairly high level of congruence in husbands' and wives' coping and the tendency to use more problem-focused strategies. These couples favored a number of coping strategies, particularly positive problem solving and rational thinking, although patients used slightly more of each strategy than their spouses did. The second cluster, with 36 couples, had a moderate degree of congruence—that is, patients and spouses were similar in their use of some strategies and not others. Both spouses and patients engaged in fairly high levels of positive problem solving. Spouses used more escape into fantasy, rational thinking, acceptance, and finding blame than did patients. Thus, although the couple solved problems together, spouses used more emotion-focused coping strategies than patients. We called this cluster *problem solvers with emotion-coping spouses.*

The third cluster, with 33 couples, although characterized by congruence, could be described as *minimalist copers*. Coping efforts by both husbands and wives were low on all strategies, and no single strategy predominated. Note that Clusters 1 and 3 are both congruent, but the intensity of their coping efforts differs.

The fourth cluster, with 30 couples, included couples whose coping styles were not congruent. Patients used a combination of distancing, rational thinking, and passive acceptance and tended *not* to use the strategies of escape or finding blame. In contrast, their healthy spouses exerted few coping efforts across the board. If any strategy predominated among spouses, it was rational thinking. We called this cluster *and the patient copes alone.*

There were no differences among the four coping clusters on any of the measures of social support: support received from the partner, support provided to the partner, and satisfaction with support. Nor were there differ-

---

[2]The seven strategies are explained as follows: *Positive problem solving* is an instrumental coping strategy with an optimistic tone. It includes items involving forward-looking, problem-focused cognitions and behaviors, such as planning for action, and reappraising the illness as a time of personal growth. *Escape into fantasy*, a cognitive avoidance strategy, describes a more passive coping style of wishing that things had happened differently and imagining a better life situation. *Distancing* describes efforts to minimize or avoid the threat and detach oneself from the emotional distress caused by the illness. *Rational thinking* reflects a calm, collected approach to managing the stressful situation. *Seeking support* involves actions to mobilize social resources for reassurance and confirmation. *Passive acceptance* includes a number of nonactions that may not make things better but prevent the situation from becoming worse. This strategy reflects the coping mode of "inhibition of action" that Lazarus (1981) described in his original paradigm but which has seldom been included in coping measures. *Finding blame* describes expressions of anger toward a person or circumstances responsible for the stresses of illness.

ences among coping clusters on any medical variables: self-reports of pain and disability, physicians' ratings of disease severity, disease activity, and disability. There was, however, a consistent and meaningful pattern of cluster differences in the couples' *subjective* experience of the illness. Couples in Cluster 1, the *effortful partnerships,* stood apart from couples in the other three clusters in a number of meaningful ways. Patients in this cluster had greater levels of depressive symptoms than patients in any of the other three clusters, with half having CES-D scores indicative of clinical depression (> 16; Radloff, 1977). Similarly, spouses perceived a much greater degree of stress in their lives than did spouses in the other clusters, particularly interpersonal stress with family and friends, illness intrusions (ways in which the partner's illness intruded into their daily lives), and caregiver burden.

These differences suggest the subtle influence of the social context on couples' coping. Patients in Cluster 1 were more distressed than patients in any other cluster, and their spouses reported a greater degree of stress. Adopting a traditional stress and coping model, we might conclude that the problem-focused efforts of these couples may have been insufficient to manage the ongoing burdens of pain and increasing disability and that the efforts by these couples to improve their situation may have left them feeling worse. Perceiving the ineffectiveness of their coping efforts, they may have tried many different types of coping strategies, also without success (Aldwin & Revenson, 1987). Either the indiscriminate use of every strategy within their repertoire led to poorer adaptive outcomes or emotional distress led these couples to try every coping strategy they could think of in an attempt to manage that distress. Although the base rate of seeking counseling was low in the full sample (approximately 23% of patients and 19% of spouses), the majority of these individuals tended to be in Cluster 1. Couples in this cluster may have been at the stage of confronting the meaning of the illness for their lives, and this may have (temporarily) heightened their emotional distress. Or, these couples may have been struggling to use active coping strategies to control a situation that was beyond their control, contributing to their emotional distress.

One other finding suggests yet another interpretation of the data. Patients and spouses in Cluster 1 had higher scores on a measure of personal growth developed to assess the positive outcomes of illness (Felton & Revenson, 1984). Thus, despite their distress, these actively coping couples were able to reappraise their illness in a more positive light and could see benefits from their struggle. Thus, contextual coping analyses may reveal a resilience that may not be apparent from approaches that examine the effect of individual-level coping strategies on individual-level outcome measures.

The less vigorous coping efforts of the three less distressed clusters may have reflected a coping response that was appropriate to the appraisal level of illness-related stress. This is consistent with Lazarus' stress and coping paradigm, emphasizing the importance of psychological appraisal processes and the situation specificity of coping (Lazarus, 1999; Lazarus & Folkman, 1984). With long-term, non-life-threatening illness and effective treatment, perceptions of illness stress may lessen or stabilize over time or couples may learn to accommodate to the vicissitudes of the illness.

Thus, dissimilar coping styles within a couple do not necessarily signal a greater level of psychological or marital problems. It is likely that the partners' different modes of coping did not cancel each other out but complemented each other, producing a wider repertoire of coping options. The question of whether the fit between husbands' and wives' coping is a greater predictor of adjustment than simply knowing which strategies were used remains unanswered; couples in one cluster characterized by high similarity were highly distressed, whereas in another cluster they were not.

These data emphasize the importance of understanding couples' life context and *their perceptions of it* as they cope with a serious illness. Coping seems less dependent on the objective circumstances of the illness and more on the couple's integration of those circumstances into their life. For example, although features of the medical context did not differentiate couples' coping patterns, the experience of pain or disability spilled over to the distress experienced by the healthy spouse.

Expanding These Approaches

All three approaches to couple-level coping provide evidence that couples' coping may be substantially different from the "sum" of the individuals' coping. Putting these three approaches together leads to a transactional process model of couples' adaptation similar to those proposed in several chapters of this book, with regard to dyadic coping (see chap. 2, this volume) and interpersonal conflict and interpersonal communication (see chap. 4, this volume). These process models revolve around the dynamic interplay of each partner's reactions. The "starting point" for this interaction is arbitrary; that is, either partner may create an emotional situation to which the other responds or a particular aspect of the illness or its treatment may elicit coordinated coping efforts by husband and wife (see chap. 2, this volume, for specific examples). Appraising the degree to which some feature of the illness is stressful, each partner tries a variety of coping strategies to minimize distress and maintain family functioning. The other partner's reaction to this coping creates, over time, a set of conditions to which the "first" partner responds. The "second" partner then tries to (re)act in a way that will minimize her or his partner's distress but may instead exacerbate it. Thus, the couple's adaptation to illness can be described as a spiral or cascade whereby the patient's distress affects the spouse's coping and support provision, which affects the patient's distress and coping, which affects the spouse, and so on (see chap. 2, this volume).

Although our study provided a rich description of couples' coping patterns, it cannot answer questions about long-term coping processes. With cross-sectional data, we can see the resulting patterns of congruence or incongruence of couples' coping but not the evolution of those patterns over time. Did one spouse's choice of coping strategy change how the other spouse coped? Do partners knowingly coordinate coping efforts, whether capitalizing on similarity or complementarity, to achieve desired outcomes? Does the couple's coping become more congruent over time as ineffective strategies or strategies that impeded a partner's coping efforts are discarded and successful ones are adopted or recycled? These are the questions for the next generation of couples' coping research.

What's Gender Got to Do With It?

One key area that has been missing from research on couples' coping, as well as coping with illness, is a deliberate consideration of gender. Gender roles are a key component of intimate relationships, and our understanding of couples' coping is not complete without this dimension.

Because of funding priorities and constraints, most research on the impact of illness has focused on single diseases. However, because many diseases vary in their prevalence among men and women, many studies include respondents of only one sex, for example, women with breast cancer or arthritis, men with prostate cancer or heart disease, and if they are couples studies, they include the husbands or wives of these patients. Thus, if differences in the impact of illness on the spouse or in the efficacy of patients' coping efforts are detected across these studies, it is difficult to disentangle the influences of gender and the person's role as patient or partner. Similarly, because few studies have included both patients and their spouses and even fewer have analyzed the data taking into account the fact that these individuals are married to each other (using nonindependent statistical tests), we cannot discern whether the experience of coping with the "same" illness in the same family differs for women and men.

Existing research presents the strong impression that men and women cope with illness in extremely different ways and that women face a greater burden than men whether they are the person with the illness or the spouse caregiver. In an early study, Hafstrom and Schram (1984) compared couples in which the husband or wife had a chronic condition with couples in which neither spouse was ill. (Unfortunately, this study did not directly compare couples with ill husbands to couples with ill wives.) Compared to their counterparts in non-ill families, wives who were chronically ill did more housework (an average of 7 hours more a week!), although they spent 6 fewer hours in the labor force. There were no differences between the groups in global marital satisfaction, although women with chronic illness were less satisfied with their role performance as wives and mothers. In contrast, wives whose husbands had a chronic illness were less satisfied with their marriages than were wives in non-ill families. Compared to healthy families, wives in marriages in which the husband was ill were significantly less satisfied in many areas, including the husband's lack of understanding of their feelings, the amount of attention the husband provided, the husband's help around the house, the husband's role performance as a husband and father, the amount of time the couple spent together, and the way this time was spent. Wives of ill husbands also were less satisfied with their own role performance as mothers, but surprisingly, *not* with their performance as wives. These data suggested that women with ill husbands felt a responsibility to keep the family and home intact, but at great personal cost.

Studies of couples coping with myocardial infarction present a similar picture.[3] After a heart attack, men tend to reduce their work activities and responsibilities and are nurtured by their wives. After hospitalization, women resume household responsibilities more quickly, including taking care of other family members, and report receiving a greater amount of help from adult daughters and neighbors than from their healthy husbands. Michela (1987), interpreting data collected from 40 couples in which the husband had suffered a first heart attack during the previous year, found substantial differences in husbands' and wives' experiences:

> *His* experience is filtered through concerns about surviving and recovering from the MI with a minimum of danger or discomfort, while *her* experience is filtered through the meaning of the marital relationship to her—what the marriage has provided and, hence, what is threatened by the husband's potential death or what is lost by his disability. (p. 272)

Is this gender? Or is it as a result of being the patient versus the caregiver?

A few studies of couples coping with illness have addressed this question directly and yielded equivocal results. Baider et al. (1989) compared patients with healthy spouses for women and men separately. Female cancer patients were more distressed than wives of male cancer patients, and in separate analyses, husbands of cancer patients reported more distress than male cancer patients. Thus, couples of female cancer patients with healthy husbands showed greater distress than couples of male patients with healthy wives. Hagedoorn and her colleagues (Hagedoorn, Buunk, Kuijer, Wobbes, & Sanderman, 2000) used a similar methodology to study gender differences but found opposite results. Wives of (male) cancer patients experienced greater distress and lower quality of life than did husbands of (female) cancer patients. Yet there were no differences between male and female *patients* in distress or quality of life. They concluded that neither gender nor role status alone makes a difference, but the combination of gender and role does. Hagedoorn and her coauthors leave us with the question, "What is it about being the partner of a patient with cancer that causes more psychological distress among women than men?" (p. 240). Possible explanations include the idea that women perceive more distress than men because they spend more hours on caregiving tasks or because they are more open about sharing feelings, or that men derive more satisfaction and self-esteem from caregiving. Our research on couples with rheumatic disease, described next, attempts to understand more fully these *his* and *hers* experiences.

Gender Differences in Marital Coping Processes Among Couples With Rheumatic Disease

Most research on psychological adjustment to rheumatic disease has focused on the patient's experience, and the majority of patients are women. Rheumatic diseases have a higher prevalence among women (approximately

---

[3]It is important to note that the majority of studies sample male patients and female spouses.

75%), and research suggests that there are meaningful gender differences in the patterning of disease, the experience of symptoms, and how patients cognitively appraise their symptoms (Danoff-Burg & Revenson, 2000; DeVellis, Revenson, & Blalock, 1997; Majerovitz & Revenson, 1994; Revenson & Danoff-Burg, 2000).

We return to the study of 113 married couples with rheumatic disease described earlier in this chapter to explore questions of gender. In all analyses, the couple is the unit of analysis. In some analyses, couples in which the husband is ill are compared with couples in which the wife is ill; in other analyses these couples are compared with an age- and income-matched comparison sample of 37 "healthy" couples in which neither spouse was diagnosed with a chronic illness.

GENDER DIFFERENCES IN COPING. Independent sample t tests were used to compare frequency of use of particular coping strategies among couples in which the wife had rheumatic disease and couples in which the husband had rheumatic disease. Few statistically significant differences were found. Female patients used escape into fantasy and seeking support to a greater extent than male patients; female spouses used more passive acceptance than male spouses.

We also determined the proportion of couples in each cluster in which the wife versus the husband was ill. Although the chi-square statistic was not significant, $\chi^2 = 3.158$ ($df = 3$), $p = .37$, the proportion of women patients in each cluster looked different: In Cluster 1, the effortful partnerships, there were six times as many couples in which the wife versus the husband had rheumatic disease. In contrast, this ratio was 2:1 in Cluster 2, 3:1 in Cluster 3, and 4:1 in Cluster 4. (The matching of the number with the cluster number is coincidental.) Thus, it seems that the pattern of couples coping that we found may be shaded by gender.

GENDER DIFFERENCES IN ADJUSTMENT. A second question involved the relative levels of psychosocial adjustment experienced by patients and their spouses and whether these outcomes varied by the patient's gender. We examined three measures of psychological adjustment (depression, psychological distress, and psychological well-being) and two measures of marital adjustment (martial satisfaction and sexual satisfaction) using a 2×2 mixed model analysis of variance with partner status (patient or spouse) as a within-couple source of variance and patient gender (male vs. female) as the between-couples factor. In this way, we could examine gender differences among patients and spouses and whether there was an interaction between patient status and gender.

Women had significantly higher scores than men on the depression, psychological distress, and sexual dissatisfaction scales (Majerovitz & Revenson, 1994). This suggests that gender has an influence on adjustment, regardless of whether one is the person with rheumatic disease or the partner of someone with rheumatic disease. However, there were a number of interesting interactions between gender and patient status. Comparing the four groups (female patients, male patients, female spouses, and male spouses), female patients had the highest levels of depression and male patients the lowest. In fact, female patients were the only group to approach the cutoff score of 16 on the CES-D (Radloff, 1977), which denotes clinical depression. Mirroring this effect, female patients had the lowest well-being scores and male patients the highest. Although there was not a significant interaction effect for marital satisfaction, there was a main effect for patient status: Patients (male and female) reported greater marital satisfaction than their healthy spouses did.

We were intrigued by the fact that female patients seemed worse off (psychologically) than male patients.[4] This mirrors the literature on sex differences in depression in the general population. We wondered if this difference might be attributed to the fact that women in this sample had more severe disease; however, there were no differences between female and male patients in physician-rated disease severity or activity or in patients' self-reports of functional ability. We then turned to other psychological explanatory variables.

GENDER DIFFERENCES IN SOCIAL SUPPORT. The provision of social support is an important aspect of couples' coping (see chaps. 4 & 7, this volume; Lyons et al., 1998). In a study of women with rheumatoid arthritis and their spouses (Revenson & Majerovitz, 1990), a number of wives of ill men confided that they had lessened their own requests for emotional support for fear of increasing their ill husbands' distress. This reflects the coping strategy of *protective buffering* described in Coyne and Smith's (1991, 1994) study of couples coping with the husband's myocardial infarction.

We hypothesized that gender differences in adjustment may reflect caregiver burden and the degree to which female and male patients feel supported by their partners. We asked about a number of dimensions of support: positive emotional support, problematic (negative) support, and satisfaction with the support received. We asked husbands and wives about the degree to which they received positive and problematic support from their partners, the degree to which they gave positive and negative support to their partners, and the degree to which they were satisfied with the instrumental and emotional support received from their partners.

Contrary to predictions, there were no differences between male and female patients' reports of the positive or problematic support they received. However, there were significant differences between male and female *spouses*: Husbands of ill women reported receiving more positive support than wives of ill men. In contrast to this finding, wives of ill men reported receiving more problematic support from their partners than did husbands of ill wives. There were no differences among men and women overall (well or ill) in the amount of positive or problematic support that they reported providing to their partner.

Although there were no gender differences in received support, these findings suggest that men and women with rheumatoid arthritis were *providing* very different levels of support to their spouse. Male spouses reported receiving higher levels of support from their ill wives than wives reported receiving from their ill husbands, indicating that the chronically ill wives in this sample were coping with their own illness while continuing to provide

---

[4]It is possible that male patients showed psychological deficits on dimensions of mental health that we did not measure, for example, alcohol or substance abuse.

social support to their husbands. In contrast, ill husbands were not providing comparable levels of support to their wives. Perhaps the chronically ill men in this sample reduced their own burden by focusing more on themselves and less on supporting their partner, whereas the women continued to care for husbands and other family members despite their illness. This is congruent with Michela's (1987) study of the experience of myocardial infarction, described earlier.

Ill wives and their husbands were equally satisfied with the instrumental and emotional support they received from each other. However, there was a large discrepancy between ill husbands and *their* wives: Ill husbands were extremely satisfied and their wives were extremely dissatisfied. In fact, wives of ill men were the least satisfied of all respondents with the instrumental and emotional support they received from their partner. If ill husbands were indeed providing less support to their wives as they focused on their own illness, as suggested above, this would explain the discrepancy in support satisfaction.

Although the women and men in this study differed on indices of psychological and marital adjustment, these differences were not a result of gender differences in coping strategies. Moreover, there was an interaction between gender and whether one is the person with rheumatic disease or the spouse of a person with rheumatic disease. The findings offer only a partial explanation for the gender differences found in psychosocial adjustment—that is, they do not explain the fact that women with rheumatic disease have higher depression scores than men with rheumatic disease—scores that approach the cutoff point for diagnosing clinical depression. It seems that male patients' low levels of depression, high levels of well-being, and high levels of sexual satisfaction may be a reflection of their high satisfaction with the support provided by their wives. The significant differences lie in perceptions of spousal support (e.g., satisfaction). Men with rheumatic disease may perceive a great deal of support and caregiving from their wives that women with rheumatic disease do not.

Reconceptualizing the Link Between Coping and Support With a Dyadic-Coping Framework: The Division of Household Labor

A number of sociological studies have documented a gender gap in the sharing of household responsibilities by women and men (Hochschild, 1989). Even with the growing proportion of women in the paid labor force, women spend an average of 15 hours more a week on household responsibilities than do men. This gender inequity was described as having important implications for the mental health of women juggling careers and family life.

The notion of a gender inequity in household responsibilities is relevant to coping processes among couples living with a chronic physical illness. If one conceives of the family as an open system, when one partner becomes ill or disabled there is a need for the family to adapt. Daily routines must be adjusted, roles restructured, and long-established patterns of family activities rearranged. As Pearlin and Turner (1987, p. 148) have written, "disruptive events acquire much of their stressful character not by their own direct impact but by disrupting and dislocating the more *structured* [italics added] elements of peoples' lives."

Coping with chronic illness requires a restructuring of household responsibilities, but we hypothesize that the nature of this restructuring differs when the wife or husband is ill: In marriages in which women are ill, we expect there will be a narrowing of the gender gap in the division of household labor; that is, men will pick up more of the ongoing household responsibilities. In contrast, in marriages in which the husband is ill, women will add even more responsibilities.

We tested these hypotheses in our sample of 113 married couples with rheumatic disease (described earlier in this chapter) that also included an age-matched comparison sample of 37 couples without a chronic illness. We asked husbands and wives (separately) about the division of household labor on 14 different household tasks. Some of these tasks were traditionally female (e.g., doing dishes), others were traditionally male (e.g., car maintenance), and yet others were ambiguous ("household finances"). For each task, respondents were asked to divide 100% into the proportion of the task that they did, that their spouse did, and that was done by other help (either family members or paid help). To examine whether the distribution of household labor differed among couples in which the wives are ill, couples in which the husbands are ill, and healthy comparison couples, we used a nonparametric statistic, the median test, which produces a chi-square statistic.

A Gender Gap in the Division of Household Labor

A gender gap in the division of household labor was apparent across the full sample of 150 couples. For most tasks, wives did over half of the work; in most cases, they did even more, and there was good agreement in these estimates between husbands and wives.[5]

Our first hypothesis addressed whether the division of household labor shifts when wives are ill and moves toward greater gender equity. There were significant differences among couples on most household tasks: For 10 of the 14 tasks, the median test was significant for the proportion of work done by the wife, and for 3 of those tasks, the median test also was significant for the proportion of work done by the husband. Wives with rheumatic disease did a significantly smaller proportion of tasks than healthy comparison wives or wives of ill husbands. Level of functional disability was inversely correlated with this decrease: that is, more disabled women did even less household work. Thus, women with rheumatic disease relinquished or were relieved of some of their household responsibilities, particularly when disability was more severe.

However, the nonsignificant median tests are informative with regard to gender. There were no significant differences among women across the three types of couples for the tasks of cooking, doing dishes, social planning, and domestic finances. Women with rheumatic disease did no less of the daily cooking or dishes as compared to healthy wives (either in couples in which the

---

[5]This finding is replicated whether we use the husband's or wife's responses about the division of labor or an average of the two. The greatest amount of disagreement was in the areas of child care and car maintenance.

husband is ill or in healthy couples); women did about two thirds of the social planning; and husband and wives in all three types of couples shared responsibility equally for domestic finances.

The second part of the hypothesis predicted not only a shift in the pattern of women's work among couples in which the wife has a chronic illness but a move toward greater gender equity. This part of the hypothesis was only partially supported and differed by type of task. For some tasks, such as *running errands* and *grocery shopping*, husbands picked up the slack, increasing their proportion of work done. For the tasks of *doing laundry and heavy cleaning*, the decrease in work by ill wives was filled by a combination of the husband doing more and using outside help (either paid help or unpaid family members).

In contrast, for the tasks of *child care* and *routine cleaning*, husbands did not increase their contribution. Instead, couples relied on other help (either paid or family help) to compensate for the ill wives' decrease. For example, ill wives did less child care than comparison wives, but the husbands of the ill women did the same amount of child care as comparison husbands. The gap was filled by other people more often for couples with ill wives than for couples with ill husbands or comparison couples.

A different picture emerges for traditionally male tasks, such as taking out the garbage, household repairs, outside chores (e.g., mowing the lawn), and car maintenance. We found few differences between couples in which the wife was ill and healthy comparison couples. Husbands of ill wives continued to do tasks that are traditionally male. Men with rheumatic disease, however, did less than either healthy husbands or husbands of ill wives. When it came to *taking out the garbage*, wives picked up that responsibility (no pun intended). With regard to *household repairs*, wives picked up some of the work and some was done by outside help. In contrast, neither *outside chores* nor *car maintenance* became the women's responsibility; these were done by outside help.

Most of the couples appeared to be resourceful in taking some of the burden off the ill partner and in getting household chores done. This may have been possible because this sample had the financial resources to do so. The picture may be different in families with fewer economic resources.

Although there was clearly a responsiveness of the couples in our study to adjust their distribution of household responsibilities when one partner has a chronic illness, women—even those who are ill—were still responsible for many of the around-the-clock maintenance tasks such as cooking, cleaning, and child care. In a qualitative study of breast cancer patients and their husbands, Zunkel (2002) reported that many husbands felt a responsibility to pitch in with child care, particularly when the woman was unable to do so because of chemotherapy or pain. Several of the husbands described this as "taking over things," which suggests that these tasks are still seen as the wife's responsibility. The manner in which household tasks are shared even in ill couples suggests that a gender-based typology persists despite illness and that certain tasks remain forever the province of husband or wife.

This finding replicates that of national studies of healthy couples (Hochschild, 1989): Women do more of the tasks that need either daily or immediate attention and fix women's lives into a more rigid routine, such as feeding the family and attending to children's needs. This can become problematic when one has a rheumatic disease that involves severe pain, joint swelling, and symptom flares that are neither predictable, controllable, nor time limited.

These data suggest that a traditional gender-typed division of labor exists even when chronic illness affects a marriage and may reveal only the visible surface of deeper emotional issues: What should a husband and a wife contribute to a family when one person is ill or disabled? How appreciated does each feel? And how does each develop a gender strategy for coping with these issues at home? These are the underlying issues that deserve further research attention in order to increase our knowledge about the specific ways in which gender is part of couples' adaptation to illness.

Explanations for the Gender Gap

In sum, wives of ill husbands reported receiving less emotional support and more problematic spousal support and were dissatisfied with the emotional and tangible support they were receiving from their partners. Perhaps it was the feeling of never-ending responsibilities that led women caring for ill husbands to feel dissatisfied with the instrumental emotional support they were receiving from their spouses. Women who had a rheumatic disease enjoyed greater sharing of responsibilities with their husbands, but the couples also relied on outside help. In contrast, in couples in which men were ill, they did even less, and their wives added on some around-the-clock maintenance to their responsibilities, perhaps leading to feelings of burden and a lack of appreciation. It is interesting that whereas wives of ill men scored neither higher than husbands of ill women on a standardized measure of caregiver burden nor lower on a measure of marital satisfaction, the variance for the wives was extremely large on both measures, indicating extreme highs and lows.

In conclusion, couples' experience of coping with illness cannot be extricated from gender. Whether they are the patient or the caregiver, women assume a disproportionate share of the responsibilities for maintaining the family's organization and providing nurturance to family members. Gilligan (1982), among others, has noted that women tend to be socialized into caretaking roles in close relationships and are more responsive to the well-being of others. One national survey found that women were 10% to 40% more likely to support a loved one during a crisis, depending on the nature of the problem (Wethington, McLeod, & Kessler, 1987). This also points to a gross inadequacy in our current conceptions of coping: If we continue to focus only on the patient's coping efforts and the patient's relation to adjustment, we miss the critical aspects of gender. Coping with illness does not simply mean being the person diagnosed; it involves caring for family members with illness as well. With the exception of the Alzheimer's disease literature, which focuses on caregiver burden, coping has largely avoided issues of gender by avoiding issues of family-level coping.

Differing gender roles and their influence on family coping processes have implications for both family functioning and health behaviors. Whereas family coping responsibilities may be natural extensions of women's roles, they create added stress for wife caregivers. When their husbands are ill, wives do not reap the same benefits of increased caregiving and support from their husbands.

We would like to end on an optimistic note, however. Gender roles have changed over the past quarter century. Cohort studies point to less differentiation in gender roles today (Deaux & LaFrance, 1998), suggesting there may be greater flexibility for families coping with stress in the future. Current studies of chronic illness, including our own, often involve individuals in middle and old age whose early gender role socialization is likely to be different than their respective cohorts of tomorrow. Only by studying couples over the life course, and at different stages of family life, will we be able to discern whether the gender differences are due to generational effects or cohort effects.

It is important to begin to assemble a literature examining the braiding of gender with couples' adaptation to illness rather than bemoan the inadequacy of past studies. The mandate of this research would be to learn the specific ways in which gender is part of couples' adaptation to illness in order to most effectively maximize family adaptation and provide guidance to practitioners.

References

Aldenderfer, M. S., & Blashfeld, R. K. (Eds.). (1984). *Quantitative applications in the social sciences: Vol. 44. Cluster analysis.* Newbury Park, CA: Sage.

Aldwin, C. M., & Revenson, T. A. (1987). Does coping help? A re-examination of the stress-buffering role of coping. *Journal of Personality and Social Psychology, 53,* 337–348.

Baider, L., Koch, U., Eascson, R., & Kaplan De-Nour, A. (1998). Prospective study of cancer patients and their spouses: The weakness of marital strength. *Psycho-Oncology, 7,* 49–56.

Baider, L., Perez, T., & Kaplan De-Nour, A. (1989). Gender and adjustment to chronic disease: A study of couples with colon cancer. *General Hospital Psychiatry, 11,* 1–8.

Berghuis, J. P., & Stanton, A. L. (2002). Adjustment to a dyadic stressor: A longitudinal study of coping and depressive symptoms in infertile couples over an insemination attempt. *Journal of Consulting and Clinical Psychology, 70,* 433–438.

Bermas, B. L., Tucker, J. S., Winkelman, D. K., & Katz, J. N. (2000). Marital satisfaction in couples with rheumatoid arthritis. *Arthritis Care and Research, 13,* 149–155.

Coyne, J. C., & Fiske, V. (1992). Couples coping with chronic and catastrophic illness. In M. A. P. Stephens, S. E. Hobfoll, & J. Crowther (Eds.), *Family health psychology* (pp. 129–149). Washington, DC: Hemisphere Publication Services.

Coyne, J. C., Rohrbaugh, M. J., Shoham, V., Sonnega, J., Nicklas, J. M., & Cranford, J. A. (2001). Prognostic importance of marital quality for survival of congestive heart failure. *American Journal of Cardiology, 88,* 526–529.

Coyne, J. C., & Smith, D. A. F. (1991). Couples coping with a myocardial infarction: A contextual perspective on wives' distress. *Journal of Personality and Social Psychology, 61,* 404–412.

Coyne, J. C., & Smith, D. A. F. (1994). Couples coping with myocardial infarction: Determinants of patients' self-efficacy. *Journal of Family Psychology, 8,* 1–13.

Cutrona, C. E. (1996). *Social support in couples.* Thousand Oaks, CA: Sage.

Danoff-Burg, S., & Revenson, T. A. (2000). Rheumatic illness and relationships: Coping as a joint venture. In K. B. Schmaling & T. G. Sher (Eds.), *The psychology of couples and illness* (pp. 105–134). Washington, DC: American Psychological Association.

Deaux, K., & LaFrance, M. (1998). Gender. In D. Gilbert, S. T. Fiske, & G. Lindzey (Eds.), *Handbook of social psychology* (4th ed., pp. 788–827). New York: Random House.

DeLongis, A., & O'Brien, T. B. (1990). An interpersonal framework for stress and coping: An application to the families of Alzheimer's patients. In M. A. P. Stephens, J. H. Crowther, S. E.

Hobfoll, & D. L. Tennenbaum (Eds.), *Stress and coping in later-life families* (pp. 221–239). Washington, DC: Hemisphere Publication Services.

DeVellis, B. M., Revenson, T. A., & Blalock, S. (1997). Arthritis and autoimmune diseases. In S. Gallant, G. P. Keita, & R. Royak-Schaler (Eds.), *Health care for women: Psychological, social, and behavioral issues* (pp. 333–347). Washington, DC: American Psychological Association.

Felton, B. J., & Revenson, T. A. (1984). Coping with chronic illness: A study of illness controllability and the influence of coping strategies on psychological adjustment. *Journal of Consulting and Clinical Psychology, 52,* 343–353.

Folkman, S., Lazarus, R. S., Dunkel-Schetter, C., DeLongis, A., & Gruen, R. J. (1986). Dynamics of a stressful encounter: Cognitive appraisal, coping, and encounter outcomes. *Journal of Personality and Social Psychology, 50,* 992–1003.

French, J. R. P., Jr., Rodgers, W., & Cobb, S. (1974). Adjustment as person–environment fit. In G. V. Coelho, D. A. Hamburg, & J. E. Adams (Eds.), *Coping and adjustment* (pp. 316–333). New York: Basic Books.

Gilligan, C. (1982). *In a different voice: Psychological theory and women's development.* Cambridge, MA: Harvard University Press.

Gray, H., Brogan, D., & Kutner, N. G. (1985). Status of life areas: Congruence/noncongruence in ESRD patient and spouse perceptions. *Social Science and Medicine, 20,* 341–346.

Hafstrom, J. L., & Schram, V. R. (1984). Chronic illness in couples: Selected characteristics, including wife's satisfactions with and perception of marital relationships. *Family Relations, 33,* 195–203.

Hagedoorn, M., Buunk, B. P., Kuijer, R. G., Wobbes, T., & Sanderman, R. (2000). Couples dealing with cancer: Role and gender differences regarding psychological distress and quality of life. *Psycho-Oncology, 9,* 232–242.

Hagedoorn, M., Kuijer, R. G., Buunk, B. P., DeJong, G. M., Wobbes, T., & Sanderman, R. (2000). Marital satisfaction in patients with cancer: Does support from intimate partners benefit those who need it most? *Health Psychology, 19,* 274–282.

Halford, W. K., Scott, J. L., & Smythe, J. (2000). Helping each other through the night: Couples and coping with cancer. In K. B. Schmaling & T. G. Sher (Eds.), *The psychology of couples and illness* (pp. 135–170). Washington, DC: American Psychological Association.

Hochschild, A. (1989). *The second shift.* New York: Viking Penguin.

Kuijer, R. G., Ybema, J. F., Buunk, B. P., DeJong, G. M., Thijs-Boer, F., & Sanderman, R. (2000). Active engagement, protective buffering, and overprotection: Three ways of giving support by intimate partners of patients with cancer. *Journal of Social and Clinical Psychology, 19,* 256–275.

Lazarus, R. S. (1981). The stress and coping paradigm. In C. Edisdorfer, D. Cohen, A. Kleinman, & P. Maxim (Eds.), *Models for clinical psychopathology* (pp. 177–214). New York: Spectrum Medical and Scientific Books.

Lazarus, R. S. (1999). *Stress and emotion.* New York: Springer Publishing Company.

Lazarus, R. S., & Folkman, S. (1984). *Stress, appraisal and coping.* New York: Springer Publishing Company.

Lazarus, R. S., & Launier, R. (1978). Stress-related transactions between person and environment. In L. A. Pervin & M. Lewis (Eds.), *Perspectives in interactional psychology* (pp. 287–327). New York: Plenum Press.

Lepore, S. J. (1997). The social context of coping with chronic stress. In B. Gottlieb (Ed.), *Coping with chronic stress* (pp.133–160). New York: Plenum Press.

Levin, J. B., Sher, T. G., & Theodos, V. (1997). The effect of intracouple coping concordance on psychological and marital distress in infertility patients. *Journal of Clinical Psychology in Medical Settings, 4,* 361–372.

Lyons, R., Mickelson, K. D., Sullivan, M. J. L., & Coyne, J. C. (1998). Coping as a communal process. *Journal of Personal and Social Relationships, 15,* 579–605.

Lyons, R., Sullivan, M. J. L., Ritvo, P., & Coyne, J. (1996). *Relationships in chronic illness and disability.* Thousand Oaks, CA: Sage.

Majerovitz, S. D., & Revenson, T. A. (1994). Sexuality and rheumatic disease: The significance of gender. *Arthritis Care and Research, 7,* 29–34.

Manne, S. L. Alfieri, T., Taylor, K. L., & Dougherty, J. (1999). Spousal negative responses to cancer patients: The role of social restriction, spouse mood and relationship satisfaction. *Journal of Consulting and Clinical Psychology, 67,* 352–361.

Manne, S., & Glassman, M. (2000). Perceived control, coping efficacy, and avoidance coping as mediators between spouses' unsupportive behaviors and cancer patients' psychological distress. *Health Psychology, 19,* 155–164.

Manne, S. L., & Zautra, A. J. (1989). Spouse criticism and support: Their association with coping and psychological adjustment among women with rheumatoid arthritis. *Journal of Personality and Social Psychology, 56,* 608–617.

Manne, S. L., & Zautra, J. (1990). Couples coping with chronic illness: Women with rheumatoid arthritis and their husbands. *Journal of Behavioral Medicine, 13,* 327–342.

Michela, J. L. (1987). Interpersonal and individual impacts of a husband's heart attack. In A. Baum & J. E. Singer (Eds.), *Handbook of psychology and health* (Vol. 5, pp. 255–301). Hillsdale, NJ: Erlbaum.

Northouse, L. L., Templin, T., & Mood, D. (2001). Couples' adjustment to breast disease during the first year following diagnosis. *Journal of Behavioral Medicine, 24,* 115–136.

Northouse, L. L., Templin, T., Mood, D., & Oberst, M. (1995). Couples' adjustment to breast cancer and benign breast disease. *Psycho-oncology, 7,* 37–48.

O'Brien, T. B., & DeLongis, A. (1996). The interactional context of problem-, emotion-, and relationship-focused coping: The role of the big five personality factors. *Journal of Personality, 64,* 775–813.

O'Brien, T. B., & DeLongis, A. (1997). Coping with chronic stress: An interpersonal perspective. In B. Gottlieb (Ed.), *Coping with chronic stress* (pp. 161–190). New York: Plenum Press.

Pasch, L. A., & Christensen, A. (2000). Couples facing fertility problems. In K. B. Schmaling & T. G. Sher (Eds.), *The psychology of couples and illness* (pp. 241–268). Washington, DC: American Psychological Association.

Patterson, J. M., & Garwick, A.W. (1994). The impact of chronic illness on families: A family systems perspective. *Annals of Behavioral Medicine, 16,* 131–142.

Pearlin, L. I., & Turner, H. A. (1987). The family as a context of the stress process. In S. V. Kasl & C. L. Cooper (Eds.), *Stress and health: Issues in research methodology* (pp. 143–165). New York: Wiley.

Pedersen, S. A., & Revenson, T. A. (in press). Parental illness, family functioning, and adolescent adjustment: A family ecology framework. *Journal of Family Psychology.*

Pistrang, N., & Barker, C. (1995). The partner relationship in psychological response to breast cancer. *Social Science and Medicine, 40,* 789–797.

Radloff, L. (1977). The CES-D scale: A self-report depression scale for research in the general population. *Applied Psychological Measurement, 1,* 385–401.

Rankin-Esquer, L. A., Deeter, A., & Taylor, C. B. (2000). Coronary heart disease and couples. In K. B. Schmaling & T. G. Sher (Eds.), *The psychology of couples and illness* (pp. 43–70). Washington, DC: American Psychological Association.

Revenson, T. A. (1994). Social support and marital coping with chronic illness. *Annals of Behavioral Medicine, 16,* 122–130.

Revenson, T. A. (2003). Scenes from a marriage: Examining support, coping, and gender within the context of chronic illness. In J. Suls & K. Wallston (Eds.), *Social psychological foundations of health and illness* (pp. 530–559). Oxford, England: Blackwell Publishing.

Revenson, T. A., & Danoff-Burg, S. (2000). Arthritis. In A. Kazdin (Editor-in-Chief.), *Encyclopedia of psychology* (Vol. 1, pp. 240–242). Washington, DC: American Psychological Association.

Revenson, T. A., & Gibofsky, A. (1995). Marriage, social support and adjustment to rheumatic diseases. *Bulletin of the Rheumatic Diseases, 44,* 5–8.

Revenson, T. A., & Majerovitz, S. D. (1990). Spouses' support provision to chronically ill patients. *Journal of Social and Personal Relationships, 7,* 575–586.

Revenson, T. A., & Majerovitz, S. D. (1991). The effects of chronic illness on the spouse: Social resources as stress buffers. *Arthritis Care and Research, 4,* 63–72.

Rohrbaugh, M. J., Cranford, J. A., Shoham, V., Nicklas, J. M., Sonnega, J., & Coyne, J. C., (2002). Couples coping with congestive heart failure: Role and gender differences in psychological distress. *Journal of Family Psychology, 16,* 3–13.

Rose, G., Suls, J., Green, P., Lounsbury, P., & Gordon, E. (1996). Comparison of adjustment, activity, and tangible social support in men and women patients and their spouses during the six months post-myocardial infarction. *Annals of Behavioral Medicine, 18,* 264–272.

Schmaling, K. B., & Sher, T. G. (2000). *The psychology of couples and illness.* Washington, DC: American Psychological Association.

Spanier, G. B. (1976). Measuring dyadic adjustment scale: New scales for assessing the quality of marriage and similar dyads. *Journal of Marriage and the Family, 38,* 15–28.

Suls, J., Green, P., Rose, G., Lounsbury, P., & Gordon, E. (1997). Hiding worries from one's spouse: Associations between coping via protective buffering and distress in male post-myocardial infarction patients and their wives. *Journal of Behavioral Medicine, 20,* 333–349.

Thoits, P. A. (1986). Social support as coping assistance. *Journal of Consulting and Clinical Psychology, 54,* 416–423.

Tucker, J. S., Winkelman, D. K., Katz, J. N., & Bermas, B. L. (1999). Ambivalence over emotional expression and psychological well-being among rheumatoid arthritis patients and their spouses. *Journal of Applied Social Psychology, 29,* 271–290.

Veit, C. T., & Ware, J. E., Jr. (1983). The structure of psychological distress and well-being in general populations. *Journal of Consulting and Clinical Psychology, 51,* 730–742.

Wethington, E., McLeod, J. D., & Kessler, R. (1987). The importance of life events for explaining sex differences in mental health. In R. C. Barnett, L. Biener, & G. K. Baruch (Eds.), *Gender and stress* (pp. 144–155). New York: Free Press.

Zunkel, G. (2002). Relational coping processes: Couples' response to a diagnosis of early stage breast cancer. *Journal of Psycho-Oncology, 20,* 39–55.

Part III

Interventions To Enhance Dyadic Coping

8

A Model Dyadic-Coping Intervention

Kathrin Widmer, Annette Cina, Linda Charvoz,
Shachi Shantinath, and Guy Bodenmann

The high divorce rates in Europe and the United States are a major sign of the current vulnerability of intimate relationships with 30% to 50% of marriages ending in divorce (Sayers, Kohn, & Heavey, 1998). Among those who are married, a large number (25%–40%) rate their marriage as unsatisfactory or distressed (Döring, Baur, Frank, Freundl, & Sottong, 1986; Van Widenfelt, Hosman, Schaap, & Van der Staak, 1996). On the other hand, studies reveal that people consider intimate partnerships, especially marriage, as a matter of great importance to them. Statistics indicate that 95% of the population gets married at least once during their lifetime, and of those who divorce, 75% to 80% remarry (Glick, 1984). What these data suggest is a discrepancy between what people desire and how the course of their lives actually plays out.

Despite the high rates of distressed marriages, only a small percentage (about 10%) of those who are in unhappy relationships actually seek marital counseling or therapy when they are confronted with growing tensions or severe conflicts (Hahlweg & Klann, 1997). Furthermore, marital therapy is not very successful in terms of bringing about a positive resolution as it tends to be sought too late. Of couples who seek help, about 50% (39%–72%) report an improvement in the quality of their relationship in comparison to 13% to 30% of couples who receive no intervention (Hahlweg & Markman, 1988; Jacobson & Addis, 1993; Jacobson et al., 1984). When the spontaneous rate of remission is taken into consideration, the improvement rate falls to approximately 40% (Hahlweg & Markman, 1988).

Although these statistics are a motivational factor for many marital therapists in continuing their work (Jacobson & Addis, 1993), these data also can be interpreted to mean that approximately half of the couples seeking help do so too late. As a consequence, they either revert to deeply entrenched negative patterns of interaction, or sometimes, divorce. Furthermore, studies have shown a relapse rate of 30%, that is, results of the therapy were not maintained over time (Snyder, Wills, & Grady-Fletcher, 1991). The rate of spontaneous worsening ranges from 4% to11% among couples after the completion of therapy (Hahlweg & Markman, 1988; Jacobson et al., 1984). This would seem to support the idea that couples often do not seek professional help until a time when restoration of relationship satisfaction through therapy is no longer possible.

In contrast, studies conducted concerning the effectiveness of *preventive* interventions have shown that by teaching important competencies at an early stage in a relationship, the risk of deterioration of the quality and stability of a relationship may be reduced, thereby reducing the risk of divorce (Hahlweg, Markman, Thurmaier, Engl, & Volker, 1998; Hahlweg, Thurmaier, Engl, Eckert, & Markman, 1993; Markman, Renick, Floyd, Stanley, & Clements, 1993; Thurmaier, Engl, Eckert, & Hahlweg, 1992). However, there is some disagreement about the effectiveness of preventive interventions for relationship distress. In general, these types of programs may work in the short term, but the programs have not been shown to produce lasting changes in relationships (Bradbury & Fincham, 1990). They tend to be more effective in preventing problems at the start of a relationship when people are still happy and are not particularly effective for those who have been married for a long time and where distress has already set in (Kaiser, Hahlweg, Fehm-Wolfsdorf, & Groth, 1998; Van Widenfeldt et al., 1996). Furthermore, most of these programs focus exclusively on communication and seek to foster communication skills. The theoretical orientations of these programs are either humanistic (e.g., the Conjugal Relationship Enhancement Program, Guerney, 1977; the Minnesota Couples Communication Program, Miller, Nunnally, & Wackman, 1975) or cognitive–behavioral (e.g., the Prevention and Relationship Enhancement Program, Markman, Floyd, Stanley, & Jamieson, 1984; Markman et al., 1993; Ein Partnerschaftliches Lernprogramm, Hahlweg et al., 1998).

Couples Coping Enhancement Training (CCET)[1] is an innovative program for teaching couples effective coping strategies to deal with various types of stress throughout the course of their relationships. It was developed in Switzerland by Bodenmann (1997) and has been implemented with about 300 couples in Switzerland and Germany. In this chapter, we describe the theoretical foundations of the CCET, the major components and structure of the program, and empirical findings demonstrating the effectiveness of the training.

Couples Coping Enhancement Training

Couples Coping Enhancement Training, or CCET, is the first marital distress prevention program to integrate cognitive–behavioral approaches with theories of stress and coping, thereby distinguishing it from all other marital distress prevention programs to date. One of the main aims of the CCET is to strengthen the coping competencies of *both* partners by strengthening dyadic communication and dyadic coping.

Dyadic coping refers to the way couples cope together, either by supporting each other or by jointly addressing stressful situations that affect them both (see chap. 2, this volume, for a full description of the theoretical model underlying this program). Dyadic coping is an important predictor of marital

---

[1]This program is known in German as *Freiburger Stresspräventionstraining für Paare* (FSPT, Bodenmann, 2000a).

quality, marital development, and marital outcomes, as it helps partners to deal more effectively with everyday stressors that can overload their individual coping resources. Dyadic coping can reduce the negative impact of stressors in daily life and strengthen individual and dyadic coping skills in response to these stressors. Thus it both reduces risk factors for marital problems and enhances the coping resources of the partners.

Stress diminishes the quality of marital communication considerably (Bodenmann, Perrez, & Gottman, 1996). Although many couples do not suffer from communication deficiencies in general, stressful conditions challenge couples' capabilities to communicate. Although most marital distress prevention programs address communication issues, they do not address some of the underlying reasons that cause communication to be compromised. CCET addresses couples' communication processes from twin perspectives: giving people basic information about how to communicate (which is similar to many other programs) along with giving information on how to *protect* the quality of communication when it is under threat of daily stress, with the goal of enhancing the effectiveness of their coping.

The goal of enhancing coping skills is supported by five major findings from our body of work (see chap. 2, this volume; Bodenmann, 2000b; Bodenmann & Shantinath, 2004): (a) Stress affects marital satisfaction both directly and indirectly; (b) the impact of stress on marital interaction can be moderated by adequate coping; (c) happy couples spontaneously practice positive dyadic coping more often than unhappy couples do; (d) the absence of positive dyadic coping is a major predictor of divorce; and (e) unhappy couples are less likely than happy couples to respond to each other's emotional distress signals. For example, a study by Bodenmann and Cina (2000) with 70 Swiss community-residing couples showed that both individual and dyadic coping play an important role in marital quality and stability. In a discriminant analysis using only the coping variables, 73% of the couples were correctly classified into one of three groups: satisfied married couples, unsatisfied married couples, and divorced couples. Couples who used positive coping strategies were able to communicate effectively with each other in everyday interactions as well as under stress and showed relatively stable marital quality over a period of 5 years. However, couples who used negative individual coping strategies (e.g., blaming and passivity) and negative dyadic coping skills (e.g., hostile or avoidance coping) or who used only a few positive dyadic coping skills were more likely to experience a significant decrease in marital quality over time.

The CCET encompasses six units that address the following topics: stress and coping, marital communication, problem solving, fairness and equity, and boundaries in close relationships (see Table 8.1). The theoretical background of the program encompasses social and cognitive behavioral theories (e.g., Gottman, Coan, Carrère, & Swanson, 1998; Jacobson, 1977, 1992; Karney & Bradbury, 1995; Weiss & Heyman, 1997), stress and coping theories (e.g., Bodenmann, 1995, 1997, 2000b; Kanner, Coyne, Schaefer, & Lazarus, 1981; Lazarus & Folkman, 1984; Perrez & Reicherts, 1992), and social exchange theory (e.g., Christensen & Shenk, 1991; Minuchin, 1977; Thibaut & Kelley, 1959; Walster, Walster, & Berscheid, 1978). The overall format is presented next, followed by detailed descriptions of the six modules.

Table 8.1. Description of the Modules of Couples Coping Enhancement Training

Module	Content	Goals	Methods and delivery	Duration (in hours)	Theoretical background
1	Knowledge of stress and coping	• Improve the participant's understanding of stress • Discriminate between different kinds of stress	• Overview of the topic of stress, including its causes, forms, and consequences • Enhancement of situation evaluation • Assessment of different areas of stress	2	• Stress theory of Lazarus and Folkman (1984) • Subsequent development of a situation-behavior-approach by Perrez and Reicherts (1992)

2	Improvement of individual coping	• Prevent stress by anticipating a stressful situation and preparing in advance, and improve coping during stressful event and in retrospect
		• Counter stress by building up a repertoire of pleasant events
		• Enhance the ability to cope with stress that is unavoidable
			• Cognitive and behavioral techniques, such as
			  –problem analyses
			  –activity planning
			  –self-observation
			  –time management
			  –cognitive restructuring
			  –self-instruction
			  –progressive muscle relaxation
				3.5	• Stress theory of Lazarus and Folkman (1984) and Lazarus (1986)
					• Situation-behavior-approach by Perrez and Reicherts (1992)
					• Kanner, Coyne, Schaefer, and Lazarus (1981)

3	Enhancement of dyadic coping	• Increase an understanding of the partner's stress • Enhance stress related communication • Improve overall dyadic coping skills	• Theoretical introduction • Supervised role plays	5	• Systemic, process-oriented approach to coping in couples developed by Bodenmann (1995, 1997; 2000b)

#	Module	Goals	Methods	Duration	Theoretical background / references
4	Exchange and fairness in the relationship	• Improve a couple's awareness of the importance of a fair and mutual exchange within the context of dyadic coping • Enhance the ability to detect inequality and dependence in the relationship • Improve sensitivity toward one's own needs and the needs of the partner	• Diagnostic exercises • Supervised role-playing that allows both partners to explore their needs • Guidelines regarding distance and closeness • Sensitization to the presence of overinvolvement that may be dependence or selfishness in relationships	2	• Minuchin (1977) • Olson, Sprenkle, and Russell (1979) • Thibaut and Kelley (1959) • Walster, Walster, and Berscheid (1978) • Christensen and Shenk (1991) • Jacobson (1992)
5	Improvement of marital communication	• Improve speaking and listening skills • Detect inadequate communication behavior	• Diagnostic exercises • Supervised role-playing within the framework of communication training	4	• Classical and social learning theories and their application within the context of dyads • Latest research findings on marital communication (Gottman, 1994; Gottman et al., 1998; Karney & Bradbury, 1995; Weiss & Heyman, 1997)
6	Improvement of problem-solving skills	• Strengthen the couple's mutual problem-solving skills	• Supervised role-playing of problem-solving situations within a structured five-step problem-solving approach	1.5	• Problem-solving training of D'Zurilla and Goldfried (1971) • Subsequent version adapted for couples (Jacobson, 1977; Weiss, Hops, & Patterson, 1973)

Overall Format of the Couples Coping Enhancement Training Program

The CCET program is conducted in a group format, with the groups consisting of four to eight couples. The rationale of the CCET is to strengthen personal and dyadic skills by means of skill-building exercises that focus on dyadic coping, communication, and conflict resolution. Regardless of group size, a ratio of one trainer per two couples is maintained during any exercises that involve role-playing (Modules 3–6). Standardization of the program is ensured through the use of a detailed and highly structured manual for trainers (training manual published in German by Bodenmann, 2000a; English translation in preparation).

The program lasts 18 hours, with six modules lasting 3 hours each. As it is modular, it can be offered in various formats. Typically the CCET is offered as a weekend workshop that begins Friday evening and ends Sunday evening, but it also can be conducted as a series of weekly training sessions of 3 hours each over a period of 6 weeks. Another format allows the training to be embedded in a weeklong *retreat* that combines therapy, vacation, and child care. The content and related exercises are identical in all three formats. The goals and content of each module are described next.

MODULE 1: KNOWLEDGE OF STRESS AND COPING.

Goals. The primary goals of this module are to improve the partners' understanding of stress and their ability to discriminate between different kinds of stress-provoking situations. This is accomplished through the enhancement of situation evaluation using criteria such as controllability, changeability, ambiguity, and certainty.

Content and Method of Implementation. This module offers the participants an overview of the concept of stress, including its causes, forms, and consequences. The central role that subjective understanding of a situation plays in stress perception is addressed—that is, whether each partner views the situation as threatening, damaging, demanding, or otherwise uncomfortable and how emotional reactions are related to stress perceptions. In addition to the didactic component of this module, couples are asked to assess different areas of stress in their own lives by means of a graphic scale that resembles a bar chart.

MODULE 2: IMPROVEMENT OF INDIVIDUAL COPING.

Goals. The major goal of this module is to improve the partners' coping skills during different phases of the stress process, that is, in anticipation of a stressful situation, during the stressful situation, and remembering the stress situation. In addition, this module aims to help participants recognize and build an adequate repertoire of pleasant events and to learn to reduce stress that is potentially avoidable.

Content and Method of Implementation. This module encompasses three elements: (a) preventing stress through better planning, organizing, boundary setting, and enhancing partners' ability to compromise; (b) countering stress by building up a repertoire of pleasant events, such as enjoyable activities and relaxation; and (c) learning ways of enhancing coping with stress that is unavoidable. This module draws on *traditional* cognitive and behavioral techniques adapted to stress and coping theory, including problem analysis, activity planning, self-observation, time management, cognitive restructuring, self-instruction, and progressive muscle relaxation (Beck, Rush, Shaw, & Emery, 1979; Bodenmann, 2000a; D'Zurilla & Goldfried, 1971).

MODULE 3: ENHANCEMENT OF DYADIC COPING.

Goals. The primary goals of this module are to increase an understanding of the partner's stress, enhance stress-related communication processes, and improve dyadic coping skills.

Content and Method of Implementation. Couples are first given a short introduction to stress communication in the dyadic coping process (which includes telling the partner explicitly what is going on and what kind of support is required) and dyadic coping skills (especially supportive dyadic coping, see chap. 2, this volume). Couples are trained using supervised role-playing in a process that we call *emotional stress exploration* (Bodenmann, 2000b). This involves teaching partners to recognize their emotional reactions, the reasons for their feeling stressed (e.g., criticism by an important other), and the cognitions and schemata that have been activated by the stressful situation (e.g., worthlessness, dependency on the evaluation of others, need for gratification, and importance of being loved). Partners then take turns practicing the role of the speaker and the role of the supporting partner. The speaker is allotted approximately 20 minutes for emotional stress exploration while the supporter practices active listening and can ask open-ended questions but does not give emotional or practical support.

Then the partner who has been playing the role of supporter is asked to provide supportive dyadic coping (e.g., empathy and understanding, solidarity, reframing, trust in the partner, and encouragement) reflecting the intensity of the emotional state of the partner who is disclosing her or his reasons for the stressor. In the final phase of the session, the person who role-played the stressed partner gives feedback as to how helpful this support was, how satisfied she or he was with the partner's support, and what else she or he would have wanted to receive from the partner. The entire exercise takes about 30 minutes per partner, after which the roles of speaker and supporter are reversed. At the end of each role-playing, the therapist briefly offers positive feedback to the partners about what they have done well and encourages them to focus specifically on those aspects of the role-playing that had been difficult for them, for example, listening without offering advice. During the role-playing the therapist is coaching both the speaker and the supporter and gives positive reinforcement on behavior that is compatible with the roles.

MODULE 4: EXCHANGE AND FAIRNESS IN THE RELATIONSHIP.

Goals. The goals of this module are to enhance exchange and fairness in a relationship by improving three areas: (a) a couple's awareness of the importance of a fair and mutual exchange within the context of dyadic coping; (b) enhancing the ability to detect inequality and dependence in the relationship; and (c) improving sensitivity toward one's own needs and the needs of the partner.

Content and Method of Implementation. The topics of exchange and fairness in a relationship are discussed in the context of giving and taking, acknowledging that clear boundaries that recognize both one's own needs and the needs of the partner need to be maintained. Guidelines regarding distance and closeness in the relationship also are provided. Couples are sensitized to boundary problems such as overinvolvement, dependence, or selfishness, which can affect positive dyadic coping or be caused by negative dyadic coping. Couples participate in diagnostic exercises and engage in supervised role-playing that allows them to explore their needs, boundaries, and issues of distance and closeness in their relationship.

MODULE 5: IMPROVEMENT OF MARITAL COMMUNICATION.

Goals. The major goal of this module is to improve martial communication by focusing on the speaking and listening skills of both partners. Each partner's ability to detect inadequate communication behavior is emphasized.

Content and Method of Implementation. Negative communication patterns as well as constructive communication behavior are discussed, and the importance of effective communication is emphasized. Couples then engage in short diagnostic exercises to help identify and understand dysfunctional communication within their relationship. The main activity of this module consists of supervised role-playing within the framework of communication training (Jacobson, 1977). In two role-playing activities of a half hour each, partners take turns modeling speaker and listener behavior. They learn how to express their feelings, cognitions, and wishes about the partner's bothersome behavior when they are playing the role as speaker and learn how to listen actively to the partner in the role of listener. During the role-playing, the therapist supervises both partners to prevent escalation of conflict while they are discussing a potentially hot issue.

MODULE 6: IMPROVEMENT OF PROBLEM SOLVING SKILLS.

Goals. The goals of this module are to make couples aware of the importance of constructive problem solving and strengthen their mutual problem-solving skills.

Content and Method of Implementation. Intervention methods consist of supervised role-playing of problem-solving situations within a structured six-step problem-solving approach in which couples discuss and practice ways of finding functional solutions to daily and relationship-oriented problems: (a) The couple chooses a problem and both partners describe their view and feelings about it; (b) both partners propose different solutions of the problems without judging each other; (c) both partners evaluate the different solutions and select the best one; (d) both partners decide when to start applying this solution, taking into account difficulties that might occur and how they could be handled, and they set a new date to reevaluate the solution; (e) the couple puts the solution in practice in everyday life; and (f) the couples evaluates the effectiveness of the solution. The therapist prompts and coaches the couple only to the degree that they need it.

Empirical Evidence for the Effectiveness of Couples Coping Enhancement Training

Besides the investigations with over 300 couples that have shown the important role of individual and dyadic coping to marital quality and stability, the effectiveness of the CCET program has been investigated in longitudinal studies (Bodenmann, Charvoz, Cina, & Widmer, 2001; Bodenmann, Perrez, Charvoz, Cina, & Widmer, 2002; Bodenmann, Pihet, Widmer, & Shantinath, in press). One study evaluated the effects of the program within 6 months after its completion. The second study (that is presented here) investigated long-term effects over 2 years. This study was conducted with 143 couples (73 couples in the intervention and 70 couples in the comparison group).

In this longitudinal study, data were collected at five points: 2 weeks prior to the intervention (pretest), 2 weeks after the training (posttest), 6 months after the training (first follow-up), 1 year after the training (second follow-up), and 2 years after the training (third follow-up). Data for the comparison group were obtained at corresponding times, with a period of 4 weeks between the pretest and the posttest.

Outcome data involved self-reports of change, standardized measures of marital functioning and coping, and behavioral observations. Couples completed a number of self-report scales at all time points, including scales of marital quality (PFB; Hahlweg, 1996), dyadic coping (FDCT-N; Bodenmann, 2000b), individual coping (Bodenmann, 2000b), communication behaviors, and a subscale of the dyadic adjustment scale (DAS) measuring thoughts of marital separation (Spanier, 1976). Couples also provided perceptions of change in marital quality, communication, individual coping, and dyadic coping at each assessment interval.

Couples in both the intervention and comparison groups were videotaped at home for three separate 10–15 minute segments at four of the assessment points (pretest, posttest, and 1-year and 2-year follow-ups). Couples were videotaped while engaged in the following tasks: (a) discussing a conflict topic together, (b) the woman describing an episode of a daily stress event while the man listened, and (c) the man describing an episode of a daily stress event while the woman listened. Systematic behavioral observations of dyadic communication and dyadic coping were made by independent observers. These discussions were coded using the marital communication categories as described by Gottman (1994) and the dyadic-coping categories as described by Bodenmann (2000b).

Participants were recruited by means of newspaper advertisements. Couples in the intervention group responded to an advertisement about the

CCET; the program was described as a stress prevention program for couples. Couples in the comparison group answered a newspaper advertisement for participants in a longitudinal study of predictors of marital functioning. Couples in the intervention group paid a nominal fee (equivalent to $200) in order to participate in the program. All couples—both those who answered the stress prevention program ads and those who answered the research study ads—had moderately low marital quality scores, although couples taking part in the prevention program reported lower marital satisfaction scores. These differences were statistically controlled in analyses of covariance whereby the initial scores (at pretest) were used as covariates.

Because it could be considered unethical to withhold treatment from couples who were requesting marital training, randomization to the two groups did not occur. Thus, this study represents a quasi-experimental design with a nonequivalent comparison group. A waiting list comparison group was not possible, as the duration of the study (2 years) was too long.

Couples in both the intervention and comparison groups were middle-aged (ages ranged from 22 to 60, with the mean age around 40) and had been in the relationship for approximately 14 years. Most couples were married (72% in the intervention group, 81% in the comparison group); 75% had children; and almost all (92%) were living in a common household at the time of their participation. The majority (> 60%) of the couples could be classified as being medium to highly educated along with a middle-level family income.

Our aims in evaluating the CCET were twofold: (a) to evaluate the quality of the CCET program including content and format and (b) to document the effectiveness of participating in the CCET program. In the postintervention assessment (2 weeks posttraining), most participants (88%) rated the training as being *good* or *very good* and were pleased with the personal benefits they obtained. In addition, 71% percent rated their personal benefits as *high* or *very high*. There was a tendency for women to rate the program as *very good* and for men to rate the training program as *good*.

With regard to subjective appraisals of change, couples who received CCET reported significantly greater change in marital satisfaction, dyadic communication, individual coping, and dyadic coping than did couples in the comparison group. The effect sizes of the subjective appraisals of change were strong at the 2-week posttest ($d > 1$). Although the effect sizes were not as high at later times, the results indicate that even after 1 year, medium to strong effect sizes ($d = .44–.79$) were obtained with regard to subjective ratings of change.

The Impact of Couples Coping Enhancement Training on Marital Quality and Relationship Functioning

Evidence of the effectiveness of the CCET program was indicated by significant Group × Time interactions in analyses of covariance conducted on the standardized outcome measures. Time and sex were used as within-subject factors, and the intervention condition (intervention vs. comparison group) was the between-subjects factor. Statistically significant preintervention differences between the groups on marital quality and age were statistically controlled through analyses of covariance (ANCOVAs).

MARITAL QUALITY. At both 6 months and 1 year postintervention, significant Time × Group interactions were found for the marital quality scale, the PFB (Bodenmann et al., 2001). Significant improvements for the intervention group were found for all three subscales: quarreling, tenderness, and togetherness/communication. Effect sizes for the PFB, as computed by the formula $M_{\text{INTERVENTION}} - M_{\text{COMPARISON}}$ / SD pooled, were low for men but moderate for women (see Table 8.2). In fact, significant improvement in marital quality was found at the 2-year assessment only for women in the intervention group. The effect sizes reflect moderate effects for women and rather weak changes for the men at all times of measurement.

INTERPERSONAL COMMUNICATION. Increases in positive communication within the relationship were found among women but not among men at the 2-week posttest as well as at the 6-month and 1-year follow-ups. Improvements were found in abilities to engage in problem solving, feedback to the partner, requests made to the partner, and active listening. A significant reduction in negative communication (especially whining and defensiveness) also was found. These findings suggest that women benefit more from this aspect of the training. An improvement of dyadic communication was also observed in the videotapes of the couples' communication behavior, as evidence by increased gazing, listening, and compliments and decreased criticism and interruption by both partners. Declines in defensiveness, domineering, belligerence, and withdrawal were found only for women (see Table 8.3).

INDIVIDUAL COPING. Significant Time × Group interactions were found with regard to 6 of 15 coping strategies: three functional coping behaviors

Table 8.2. Effect Sizes of Marital Quality, Coping, and Communication for Couples in the Intervention Group

Measure	Effect sizes							
	After 2 weeks		After 6 months		After 1 year		After 2 years	
	Women	Men	Women	Men	Women	Men	Women	Men
Marital quality (PFB)	.48	.31	.40	.11	.56	.26	.42	.12
• Tenderness	.33	.22	.22	.09	.48	.29	.24	.17
• Quarreling	−.31	−.32	−.41	−.21	−.37	−.14	−.26	−.11
• Communication	.45	.13	.28	−.05	.38	.14	.45	.18
Individual coping (INCOPE)								
• Functional coping	.82	.48	.74	.23	.58	.36	.54	.36
• Dysfunctional coping	−.73	−.13	−.74	−.30	−.69	−.45	−.50	.03
Dyadic coping (FDCT-N)								
• Stress communication	.34	.22	.32	.07	.16	.25	.20	.40
• Positive dyadic coping	.52	.22	.45	.12	.50	.06	.45	.15
• Negative dyadic coping	−.39	−.09	−.15	−.07	−.39	−.09	−.29	−.19
• Total of dyadic coping	.60	.31	.39	.15	.40	.25	.50	.27
Dyadic communication								
• Total dyadic communication score	.51	.13	.20	−.16	.43	.22	.26	.07

(active influence, positive self-verbalization, and information seeking) with a corresponding decrease in three dysfunctional coping behaviors (rumination, self-blaming, and negative emotional expression). There was a marginal effect (decrease) for blaming the partner. Thus, participation in the CCET is associated with improvements in individual-level functional coping and reductions in dysfunctional coping. The effect sizes were moderate for both partners but higher for women (Table 8.3).

DYADIC COPING. Clearly, changes in dyadic coping processes are the most salient outcome of the intervention. At the 2-week posttest, 6-month follow-up, and 1-year follow-up, we found significant improvements in supportive dyadic coping and common dyadic coping, along with a decline in hostile dyadic coping among the intervention group but not in the comparison group. These effects were stronger for women than men at the 1-year follow-up. These effects were not as strong at the 2-year follow-up, although the Group × Time interactions were still statistically significant. The strongest long-term effect was a reduction in hostile dyadic coping. Furthermore, compared to the comparison group, the couples in the intervention group were more satisfied with the supportive dyadic coping of their partners at both the 1- and 2-year follow-ups and considered their partner's dyadic coping as more effective and helpful at both times (Table 8.3). The observational data also found an increase in empathy–interest

Table 8.3. Effect Sizes for Observed Marital Communication and Dyadic Coping (Video Data)

	After 2 weeks		After 1 year		After 2 years	
	Women	Men	Women	Men	Women	Men
Marital communication						
Gaze	.63	1.16	.42	1.50	.47	.68
Listening	.77	.51	.88	.67	1.04	.51
Self-disclosure	.23	.27	−.16	−.27	.13	.00
Compliments	.30	.30	.57	.06	.74	.53
Affection	−.10	−.32	.39	−.30	.07	.31
Criticism	−.35	−.73	−.58	−.86	−.57	−.77
Defensiveness	−.78	−.04	−.68	−.34	−.69	−.04
Contempt	−.60	−.79	.19	.21	.15	.07
Domineering	−.69	−.71	−.57	−.13	−.54	.00
Belligerence	−.62	.41	−.14	.60	−.49	.60
Interruption	−.32	−.32	−.31	.32	−.26	−.37
Withdrawal	−.19	−.06	−.51	−.76	−.52	.00
Dyadic coping						
Empathy/interest	.60	.66	.87	.66	.45	.66
Emotion-focused supportive dyadic coping	.27	.35	−.05	.35	−.35	.35
Problem-focused supportive dyadic coping	−.03	.10	.00	.10	−.20	.10
Common dyadic coping	−.20	−.03	.32	−.03	.32	−.03
Superficial dyadic coping	−.45	−.60	−.43	−.60	−.33	−.60
Ambivalent dyadic coping	−.43	−.15	−.32	−.15	−.37	−.15

and a decrease in superficial dyadic coping in both partners, but a decrease in ambivalent dyadic coping was found only for women (Table 8.3).

Conclusion

In this chapter, we provided an overview of CCET, an innovative intervention program that focuses on the enhancement of dyadic coping resources in couples. A major feature of this program that distinguishes it from other existing marital skills training programs is the central role ascribed to dyadic coping, both in promoting marital satisfaction as well as in reducing marital distress. As stress has a negative effect on marital life (see chap. 1, this volume; Bodenmann, 2000b), it is crucial to strengthen coping resources among couples in order to help them maintain a high level of marital quality. Results on the effectiveness of the program reveal that the CCET is capable of improving marital quality and marital competencies even in couples with a low level of marital quality.

In addition to being a prevention program that emphasizes coping with stress, another aspect of CCET that distinguishes it from other marital distress prevention programs is its effectiveness with couples who have been married a long time. Data from a 2-year follow-up of CCET showed that there is an improvement in marital satisfaction, particularly among the wives of couples who had been together for a long time and were experiencing marital dissatisfaction at the time of the training (Bodenmann et al., 2001). This finding supports our view that in addition to communication skills, coping skills need to be addressed in order to help couples improve marital quality, as they are a major factor in communication deficiencies.

With regard to dyadic coping, women were more likely than men to report a higher increase of positive dyadic coping and a greater decline of negative dyadic coping. It seems noteworthy that before the training, women's level of satisfaction with their partner's support was lower than the men's satisfaction with partner support. Women's greater perception of increase in marital quality compared to that of their partner, along with their greater reports of positive dyadic coping, confirm the position of Acitelli and Antonucci (1994) that reciprocity in mutual support is of higher importance for women's satisfaction with relationships than for men's. When there is not mutual support, women tend to react with a greater decrease of marital satisfaction and well-being (Bodenmann, 2000b).

Both partners showed an increase in empathy and interest for their partner and less superficial and ambivalent dyadic coping after the training. Thus, the CCET seems to stimulate both partners to be more reciprocal in their support during stressful situations and to feel more understood and assured by their partner. This mutual increase in empathy and interest may contribute to the greater increase in marital satisfaction in women over time, as women tend to feel less understood and assured by their partner than do men (Campbell, Converse, & Rodgers, 1976; Vanfossen, 1981).

We envision that marital distress prevention programs such as the CCET will gain even more importance in the future and will be tailored for couples experiencing different types of stressors. We are aware of the interpretive limits of the results because of the lack of a strictly randomized control group, and therefore randomized studies should be conducted as a next evaluation step in different cultural contexts. Despite the limitations because of motivational factors that might have influenced the outcomes, the effect sizes indicate the program's potential efficacy and the hope for a wide range of application possibilities for the program. In our view, the CCET is ideal not only for couples starting out in their relationship but also for those who have been together for longer periods of time and who are concerned about maintaining marital satisfaction in the long run. It is especially indicated for "high risk" couples who may be facing above average levels of stress as a result of the demands of their profession (e.g., police, physicians, and corporate executives). Given our findings with regard to reducing marital distress and improving satisfaction, we think that this program will be applicable to those who have already experienced an erosion of marital quality over time from stresses brought about by common life events such as the birth of a child or loss of a job. Because it focuses on stressors external to the couple as well as on couples' interpersonal functioning, the program is met with a greater acceptance among couples who are otherwise reluctant to participate in marital therapy or marital skills training.

References

Acitelli, L. K., & Antonucci, T. C. (1994). Gender differences in the link between marital support and satisfaction in older couples. *Journal of Personality and Social Psychology, 67,* 688–698.

Beck, A. T., Rush, A. J., Shaw, B. F., & Emery, G. (1979). *Cognitive therapy of depression.* New York: Guilford Press.

Bodenmann, G. (1995). A systemic-transactional view of stress and coping in couples. *Swiss Journal of Psychology, 54,* 34–49.

Bodenmann, G. (1997). Dyadic coping—a systemic-transactional view of stress and coping among couples: Theory and empirical findings. *European Review of Applied Psychology, 47,* 137–140.

Bodenmann, G. (2000a). *Kompetenzen für die Partnerschaft* [Competencies for marriage]. Weinheim, Germany: Juventa.

Bodenmann, G. (2000b). *Stress und Coping bei Paaren* [Stress and coping in couples]. Göttingen, Germany: Hogrefe.

Bodenmann, G., Charvoz, L., Cina, A., & Widmer, K. (2001). Prevention of marital distress by enhancing the coping skills of couples: 1-year follow-up-study. *Swiss Journal of Psychology, 60,* 3–10.

Bodenmann, G., & Cina, A. (2000). Stress und Coping als Prädiktoren für Scheidung: Eine prospektive Fünf-Jahres-Längsschnittstudie [Stress and coping as predictors for divorce: A 5-year prospective longitudinal study]. *Zeitschrift für Familienforschung, 12,* 5–20.

Bodenmann, G., Perrez, M., Charvoz, L., Cina, A., & Widmer, K. (2002). The effectiveness of coping-focused prevention approach: A two-year longitudinal study. *Swiss Journal of Psychology, 61,* 195–202.

Bodenmann, G., Perrez, M., & Gottman, J. M. (1996). Die Bedeutung des intrapsychischen Copings für die dyadische Interaktion [The significance of individual coping for marital interaction]. *Zeitschrift für Klinische Psychologie, 25,* 1–13.

Bodenmann, G., Pihet, S., Widmer, K., & Shantinath, S. (in press). Improving dyadic coping among couples with low marital satisfaction: A 2-year longitudinal study. *Behavior Modification.*

Bodenmann, G., & Shantinath, S. (2004). The Couples Coping Enhancement Training (CCET): A new approach to prevention of marital distress based upon stress and coping. *Family Relations, 53,* 477–484.

Bradbury, T. N., & Fincham, F. D. (1990). Attributions in marriage: Review and critique. *Psychological Bulletin, 107,* 3–33.

Campbell, A., Converse, P., & Rodgers, W. (1976). *The quality of American life: Perceptions, evaluations, and satisfactions.* New York: Russell Sage Foundation.

Christensen, A., & Shenk, J. L. (1991). Communication, conflict, and psychological distance in nondistressed, clinic, and divorcing couples. *Journal of Consulting and Clinical Psychology, 59,* 458–463.

Döring, G., Baur, S., Frank, P., Freundl, G., & Sottong, U. (1986). Ergebnisse einer repräsentativen Umfrage zum Familienplanungsverhalten in der Bundesrepublik Deutschland 1985 [Results of a representative study of the family planning behavior in Germany]. *Geburtshilfe und Frauenheilkunde, 46,* 892–897.

D'Zurilla, T. J., & Goldfried, M. R. (1971). Problem-solving and behavior modification. *Journal of Abnormal Psychology, 78,* 107–126.

Glick, P. C. (1984). How American families are changing. *American Demographics, 6,* 20–27.

Gottman, J. M. (1994). *What predicts divorce?* Hillsdale, NJ: Erlbaum.

Gottman, J. M., Coan, J., Carrère, S., & Swanson, C. (1998). Predicting marital happiness and stability from newlywed interactions. *Journal of Marriage and the Family, 60,* 5–22.

Guerney, B. G. (1977). *Relationship enhancement.* San Francisco: Jossey-Bass.

Hahlweg, K. (1996). *Fragebogen zur Partnerschaftsdiagnostik (FPD)* [Questionnaire for the assessment of marital quality]. Göttingen, Germany: Hogrefe.

Hahlweg, K., & Klann, N. (1997). The effectiveness of marital counseling in Germany: A contribution to health services research. *Journal of Family Psychology, 11,* 410–421.

Hahlweg, K., & Markman, H. J. (1988). Effectiveness of behavioral marital therapy: Empirical status of behavioral techniques in preventing and alleviating marital distress. *Journal of Consulting and Clinical Psychology, 56,* 440–447.

Hahlweg, K., Markman, H. J., Thurmaier, F., Engl, J., & Volker, E. (1998). Prevention of marital distress: Results of a German prospective longitudinal study. *Journal of Family Psychology, 12,* 543–556.

Hahlweg, K., Thurmaier, F., Engl, J., Eckert, V., & Markman, H. J. (1993). Prävention von Beziehungsstörungen [Prevention of relationship disorders]. *System Familie, 6,* 89–100.

Jacobson, N. S. (1977). Problem-solving and contingency contracting in the treatment of marital discord. *Journal of Consulting and Clinical Psychology, 45,* 92–100.

Jacobson, N. S. (1992). Behavioural couple therapy: A new beginning. *Behaviour Therapy, 23,* 493–506.

Jacobson, N. S., & Addis, M. E. (1993). Research on couples and couple therapy: What do we know? Where are we going? *Journal of Consulting and Clinical Psychology, 61,* 85–93.

Jacobson, N. S., Follette, W. C., Revenstorf, D., Baucon, D. H., Hahlweg, K., & Margolin, G. (1984). Variability in outcome and clinical significance of behavioral marital therapy: A reanalysis of outcome data. *Journal of Consulting and Clinical Psychology, 52,* 497–504.

Kaiser, A., Hahlweg, K., Fehm-Wolfsdorf, G., & Groth, T. (1998). The efficacy of a compact psychoeducational group training program for married couples. *Journal of Consulting and Clinical Psychology, 66,* 753–760.

Kanner, A. D., Coyne, J. C., Schaefer, C., & Lazarus, R. S. (1981). Comparisons of two modes of stress measurement: Daily hassles and uplifts versus major life events. *Journal of Behavioral Medicine, 4,* 1–39.

Karney, B. R., & Bradbury, T. N. (1995). The longitudinal course of marital quality and stability: A review of theory, method, and research. *Psychological Bulletin, 118,* 3–34.

Lazarus, R. S. (1986). Puzzles in the study of daily stress. In R. K. Silbereisen, K. Eyferth, & G. Rudiger (Eds.), *Development as action in context* (pp. 39–53). Berlin, Germany: Springer Publishing Company.

Lazarus, R. S., & Folkman, S. (1984). *Stress, appraisal, and coping.* New York: Springer Publishing Company.

Markman, H. J., Floyd, F., Stanley, S., & Jamieson, K. (1984). A cognitive–behavioral program for the prevention of marital and family distress: Issues in program development and delivery. In K. Hahlweg & N. S. Jacobson (Eds.), *Marital interaction: Analysis and modification.* New York: Guilford Press.

Markman, H. J., Renick, M. J., Floyd, F. J., Stanley, S. M., & Clements, M. (1993). Preventing marital distress through communication and conflict management trainings: A 4- and 5- year follow-up. *Journal of Consulting and Clinical Psychology, 61,* 70–77.

Miller, S. M., Nunnally, E., & Wackman, D. (1975). Minnesota couples communication program (MCCP): Premarital and marital groups. In D. H. Olson (Ed.), *Treating relationships* (pp. 21–40). Lake Mills, IA: Graphic.

Minuchin, S. (1977). *Families and family therapy.* Cambridge, MA: Harvard University Press.

Olson, D. H., Sprenkle, D. H., & Russell, C. S. (1979). Circumplex model of marital and family systems: Cohesion and adaptability dimensions, family types, and clinical application. *Family Process, 18,* 3–27.

Perrez, M., & Reicherts, M. (1992). *Stress, coping and health: A situation-behavior-approach: Theory, methods, applications.* Toronto, Canada: Hogrefe & Huber.

Sayers, S. L., Kohn, C. S., & Heavey, C. (1998). Prevention of marital dysfunction: Behavioral approaches and beyond. *Clinical Psychology Review, 18,* 713–744.

Snyder, D. K., Wills, R. M., & Grady-Fletcher, A. (1991). Long-term effectiveness of behavioral versus insight-oriented marital therapy: A 4-year follow-up study. *Journal of Consulting and Clinical Psychology, 59,* 138–141.

Spanier, G. B. (1976). The measurement of marital quality. *Journal of Sex and Marital Therapy, 5,* 288–300.

Thibaut, J. W., & Kelley, H. H. (1959). *The social psychology of groups.* New York: Wiley.

Thurmaier, F., Engl, J., Eckert, V., & Hahlweg, K. (1992). Prävention von Ehe- und Partnerschaftsstörungen EPL (Ehevorbereitung—Ein Partnerschaftliches Lernprogramm) [Prevention of distress in marital and close relationships]. *Verhaltenstherapie, 2,* 116–124.

Vanfossen, B. (1981). Sex differences in the mental health effects of spouse support and equity. *Journal of Health and Social Behavior, 22,* 130–143.

Van Widenfelt, B., Hosman, C., Schaap, C., & Van der Staak, C. (1996). The prevention of relationship distress for couples at risk: A controlled evaluation with nine-month and two-year follow-up results. *Family Relations, 45,* 156–165.

Walster, E., Walster, G. W., & Berscheid, E. (1978). *Equity: Theory and research.* Boston: Allyn & Bacon.

Weiss, R. L., & Heyman, R. E. (1997). A clinical overview of couples interactions. In W. K. Halford & H. J. Markman (Eds.), *Clinical handbook of marriage and couples interventions* (pp. 13–41). New York: Wiley.

Weiss, R. L., Hops, H., & Patterson, G. R. (1973). A framework for conceptualizing marital conflict, a technology for altering it, some data for evaluating it. In L. A. Hamerlynck, L. C. Handy, & E. J. Mash (Eds.), *Behavior therapy in the psychiatric setting* (pp. 331–364). Baltimore: Williams & Wilkins.

9

Enhancing Dyadic Coping During a Time of Crisis: A Theory-Based Intervention With Breast Cancer Patients and Their Partners

Karen Kayser

Patient: Coping to him and me is that we talk about the breast cancer and we deal with it.
Patient's Husband: We share decisions; we share the research. One of us isn't running off saying, "This is what I'm doing. I don't care—it's my disease." It's shared—it's a *we-disease*.
Patient: . . . that was the most impressive thing he said to me. He calls it a we-disease. He just said it to me a couple of weeks ago.
Patient's Husband: Isn't that what it is?
Patient: It is, but it doesn't mean that everyone thinks that way.

It is an accepted fact in social science research that women with breast cancer do not cope with their illness in isolation but, instead, within the context of their interpersonal relationships. Although the relational context is recognized as important for the patient's adjustment to the illness, most studies of cancer patients and their partners continue to analyze coping as an individual phenomenon. Recently, there have been empirical investigations that examine how couples cope *together* with the cancer diagnosis. In these studies, the unit of analysis has become the couple, which allows for a more accurate description of dyadic coping processes, including those aspects of a couple's relationship that enhance coping by the partners. Likewise, several psychosocial interventions have begun to use a couples approach. The aims of this chapter are threefold. First, I review research studies that support the proposition that relationship factors such as partner support and dyadic coping moderate the stress associated with the breast cancer diagnosis and treatment. Second, I present an overview of the empirically tested psychosocial interventions that currently exist for breast cancer patients. Finally, I describe the Partners in Coping Program (PICP), a new preventive psychosocial intervention for couples coping with breast cancer, and present preliminary findings on its effectiveness.

This research was supported by a grant from the Massachusetts Department of Public Health Breast Cancer Research Program.

Breast Cancer as a Stressor for Patients and Their Partners

Types of Stress Experienced With Breast Cancer

Women[1] with breast cancer and their partners are challenged by a series of *medical, instrumental, social, emotional, and existential* demands that can subject them to considerable stress (Chesler & Barbarin, 1986; Germino, Fife, & Funk, 1995; Hannum, Giese-Davis, Harding, & Hatfield, 1991; Manne, 1998; Morse & Fife, 1998; Northouse, 1989, Northouse, Templin, Mood, & Oberst, 1998). These stresses can be classified as direct dyadic stress in that one partner has the disease but the other partner is coping with stress at the same time (see chap. 2, this volume). Therefore, breast cancer can subject the *healthy* partner or spouse to considerable stress.

MEDICAL STRESSORS. At the time of diagnosis, there are medical stresses associated with negotiating a complex healthcare organization, reading and processing a wealth of medical information, and making treatment decisions. Treatments, such as surgery, which alter a woman's body image and sexuality, and postsurgical chemotherapy with its possible side effects of nausea, vomiting, fatigue, and hair loss, challenge a couple's ability to cope. There are concerns about leaving family or work unattended in order to enter the hospital, attend clinic visits, or deal with being ill from the chemotherapy.

INSTRUMENTAL STRESSORS. While managing these medical demands, couples are dealing with the basic tasks of daily living such as household work, childcare, elder care, and outside employment. Couples need a coordinated and cooperative approach to deal with the multiple instrumental demands of carrying out the work of the family. In most families, especially families with traditional role expectations, women usually do many of the practical and nurturant tasks (Rolland, 1994). Given the patient's physical limitations, the couple needs to develop a division of labor that spreads some of the instrumental demands around in order to conserve and use family energies effectively.

SOCIAL STRESSORS. This type of stress may be experienced by the couple as they disclose the cancer diagnosis to friends and family (Chesler & Barbarin, 1986). Decisions about whom to tell and from whom to elicit support need to be made. It is not unusual for some social relationships to change, either becoming closer or more distant. Feeling uncomfortable with the diagnosis, some friends may treat the couple differently and avoid social contact. Social and recreational activities may change for the couple as they need to spend more time at home or desire to be with each other.

EMOTIONAL STRESSORS. The *emotional stressors* of breast cancer have been well documented in the research literature. Cross-sectional studies have found high levels of depression, sadness, and anxiety (Anderson, 1994; Massie & Holland,

---

[1]Although men can also be diagnosed with breast cancer, cases of male patients account for about 1% of all breast cancers (American Cancer Society, 2002). Given this low rate among men, the empirical research on male patients with breast cancer is very sparse. Therefore, the focus in this chapter is on female patients.

1991; Meyerowitz, 1986; Spiegel, 1995, 1996). Anxiety and depression can persist for a significant number of breast cancer patients even 1 year after the diagnosis (Omne-Ponten, Holmberg, & Sjoden, 1994). The behavioral manifestations of these emotions can include insomnia, inability to concentrate, loss of appetite, greater use of alcohol and tranquilizers, thoughts of suicide, sexual dysfunction, and disruption of daily activities (Irvine, Brown, Crooks, Roberts, & Browne, 1991; Meyerowitz, 1983). Although only a small percentage of women with breast cancer may actually meet the *DSM–IV* diagnosis of posttraumatic stress disorder (PTSD), breast cancer is often considered a traumatic event (Baum & Posluszny, 2001). Breast cancer patients are more likely than the general population to experience symptoms of PTSD including repeated, disturbing memories and dreams of their cancer treatment, fears of recurrence, fears of death, and physical reactions when something reminds them of cancer treatment or their experience with cancer (Cordova et al., 1995). Typically, distress increases during the first year after the cancer diagnosis, but then patients often return to a premorbid level of emotional well-being (Charles, Sellick, Montesanto, & Mohide, 1996; Greenberg et al., 1994; Kayser & Sormanti, 2002; Polinsky, 1994; Stanton & Snider, 1993).

The emotional well-being of the healthy partner will be affected by the realities and perceptions of the disease as it affects their ill partner, their own lives, and their relationships (Slaikeu, 1990). During the early phase of the illness, anxiety, depression, feelings of inadequacy about their ability to help their partners through the crisis, and somatic preoccupations are common (Sabo, 1990). Husbands commonly suffer from postsurgical distress and mood disturbance after a wife's mastectomy (Maguire, 1981; Northouse & Swain, 1987) and express problems concerning sexual intimacy (Harwood & O'Connor, 1994; Sabo, 1990; Schain, 1988). Many husbands feel unprepared to cope with their own emotional reaction to breast cancer and its treatment, and experience similar levels of difficulty in making psychosocial adjustment as do their ill wives (Oberst & James, 1985; Walker, 1997). The demands of a woman's chronic illness can affect her husband's level of depression and his perception of marital adjustment (Lewis, Woods, Hough, & Bensley, 1989).

EXISTENTIAL STRESSORS. A final type of stress that is experienced by couples is existential. This stress involves issues around the meaning and purpose of life, the unfairness of the disease, and the possibility of death. The fundamental fear of death associated with cancer is well described by Nuehring and Barr (1980). However, little is known about how a couple copes with existential issues associated with a cancer diagnosis. For example, how do they make meaning of the illness in their lives? Couples' efforts to make sense of their experience suggest an attempt to create order out of the chaos they are experiencing and perhaps to gain some sense of control over the uncontrollable as they cope with breast cancer (Collins, Taylor, & Skokan, 1990; Nadeau, 1998; Taylor, 1983).

The Role of Partner Support in Adaptation to Breast Cancer

Women report better emotional adjustment after a diagnosis of breast cancer if their husbands or partners are highly supportive (Kayser & Sormanti, 2002; Kayser, Sormanti, & Strainchamps, 1999; Lichtman, Taylor, & Wood, 1987;

Northouse, Templin, & Mood, 2001; Primomo, Yates, & Woods, 1990). Furthermore, support from family and friends can significantly affect the mental and physical functioning of women with breast cancer over a course of several years after the diagnosis (Helgeson, Snyder, & Seltman, 2004). Typically, a woman's husband or intimate partner is the first person from whom support is sought (Cutrona, 1996). Although women may seek support from other sources (friends, neighbors, and coworkers), these alternative sources cannot compensate for the lack of marital support when coping with a life-threatening illness (Cutrona). For example, in a comprehensive study of 1,715 women with breast cancer, the support provided by friends and family was not perceived by the women to be as important as support received from a spouse or significant other (Penman et al., 1986). What appeared to be most important were the women's perceptions that comfort, concern, positive regard, affection, and help with problems would be available from people close to them. Marital status by itself was not an important predictor of adjustment, which supports the idea that merely being married is not enough to cope successfully with cancer.

The quality of support a woman receives from her partner is associated with psychological well-being and positive adaptation (Northouse, Dorris, & Charron-Moore, 1995; Pistrang & Barker, 1995). Helgeson and Cohen (1996) examined several dimensions of social support and found that emotional support appears to be the most important for the psychological well-being of breast cancer patients. They defined emotional support as "the verbal and nonverbal communication of caring and concern. It includes listening, 'being there,' empathizing, reassuring, and comforting" (p. 135). They further described its benefits as permitting the expression of feelings that may reduce distress and lead to an improvement of interpersonal relationships, thus providing an element of meaning to the disease experience. Cancer patients have identified emotional support as the most helpful kind of support from partners and informational support as the most helpful from health care professionals (Dakof & Taylor, 1990; Dunkel-Schetter, 1984; Neuling & Winefield, 1988). Other studies have also shown that the most frequently reported *unhelpful behavior* is the failure to provide emotional support: "Avoiding the patient, minimizing the patient's problems, and forced cheerfulness all keep the patient from discussing the illness. The availability of someone with whom the patient can discuss illness-related concerns is central to the concept of emotional support" (Helgeson & Cohen, p. 137).

Other investigations also reveal significant relationships between emotional support and psychosocial adjustment of breast cancer patients. In a study of 86 women with advanced breast cancer, Bloom and Spiegel (1984) found that emotional support was related to the women's decreased use of *avoidance coping*, that is, socially isolating themselves. In turn, the decreased use of avoidance coping was associated with less emotional distress, fewer feelings of powerlessness, and improved self-concept. The association between emotional support and adjustment has been found in both correlational and longitudinal studies. The longitudinal studies imply a causal relationship between perceived emotional support and emotional adjustment (Kayser & Sormanti, 2002; Northouse, 1989), positive coping strategies (Bloom, 1982), and reduced distress and survival (Ell, Nishimoto, Mediansky, Mantell, & Hamovitch, 1992).

There also is evidence that support provided *by* breast cancer patients plays a critical role in their partner's adjustment. In a longitudinal study of 121 husbands of breast cancer patients, marital support was a significant predictor of both emotional and physical adjustment (Hoskins et al., 1996). Husbands who were dissatisfied with the emotional support they received experienced significantly more negative emotions, such as worry, tension, and uneasiness, which continued throughout the 12-month study period. In contrast, husbands who felt supported by their (ill) wives experienced fewer negative emotions and a sense of psychological well-being, such as enjoyment in talking with others, finding work and other things of interest, and feeling needed and useful. In addition, husbands' physical symptoms were related to unmet needs for support as late as 12 months after the patient's surgery.

Coping Behaviors Associated With Adjustment to Breast Cancer

According to Bodenmann's model of dyadic coping (see chap. 2, this volume), breast cancer can be seen as a dyadic stressor, that is, a stressor that affects both partners. As such, coping needs to be viewed as a way that the couple manages the stress together. Dyadic coping is defined as a stress management process in which partners either ignore or react to each other's stress signal in order to maintain or return to homeostasis (in this case, a preillness level of well-being) on the individual level, the couple level, and the extramarital level. Each partner's well-being depends on the other's well-being as well as on the couple's ability to use resources in the social environment during the stress management process. Assuming that both partners are willing to invest in the relationship and are committed to the relationship, they will be motivated to help each other deal with stressful encounters. Research on couples coping with breast cancer reveals that the coping strategies used by one partner can affect the other partner's adjustment to the stress of the illness. Wives' adjustment to breast cancer has been associated with their husbands' use of external control–resignation types of coping (Hannum et al., 1991), husbands' use of more problem-focused coping (Ptacek, Ptacek, & Dodge, 1994), and husbands' use of active engagement coping strategies (Kuijer et al., 2000). Cancer patients were more likely to feel distressed when their husbands used wishful thinking (Ptacek et al., 1994) and were overprotective toward them (Kuijer et al., 2000).

Similarly, breast cancer patients' coping strategies also impact their husbands' adjustment. Hannum et al. (1991) found that husbands' distress was related to a combination of their own and their wives' coping behavior. In particular, husbands' denial and observed confronting behavior and wives' higher optimism were significant predictors of husbands' distress. In another study (Ptacek et al., 1994), husbands reported more relationship satisfaction and higher levels of mental health when their wives reported using more problem-focused coping and less avoidance. The wife's use of wishful thinking was inversely related to her husband's mental health (Ptacek et al., 1994). These studies illustrate the significant crossover associations between the coping reported by one spouse and the other spouse's outcomes.

Using qualitative methods, Skerrett (1998) interviewed 20 couples about their coping with breast cancer as a couple, focusing on factors such as communication, beliefs regarding illness and health, problem-solving techniques, feelings of loss and disfigurement, and other topics related to their experience. Based on the interview data, couples were categorized as either resilient or problematic. The majority of couples (85%) were seen as resilient: They had a philosophy of coping that was mutual and served as a basis for dealing with the ongoing illness demands. They strongly believed that they were *in it together* and served as each other's confidante, advisor, and sounding board. Their communication was selective in that they were sensitive of what and when they communicated in relation to the other's perceived level of reception. Most talked openly about cancer but did not allow the talk of the illness to dominate their daily living.

In contrast, there was a small cluster of "problematic" couples (15%), for whom breast cancer had a devastating impact on their lives. The illness seemed to color every aspect of their interaction. To be fair, most of these couples also were struggling with additional problems that may have created a *pileup effect* and overloaded the couple with stress. (This finding is similar to that reported by Karney, Story, & Bradbury, chap. 1, this volume, who found chronic stress to be related to marital distress.) The "problematic" couples were unable to formulate a common coping philosophy regarding the many illness demands. Their communication took the form of one of two patterns: individual retreat into withdrawal and silence or reactive, anxiety-driven, tell-all communication. These couples did not use their previous experiences of coping with stress as a guide to help them with their current coping. They struggled to find ways to understand and make meaning of the experience.

In sum, the research indicates that both the patient and partner are affected by the stress of breast cancer. How each partner copes with the multiple stressors posed by the illness, its treatment, and its meaning will affect the other partner's coping and psychosocial adjustment. The provision of support from each person significantly contributes to the individual well-being of both the patient and partner. However, as noted by Pistrang and Barker (see chap. 5, this volume), little attention in the research literature has been given to understanding the *informal helping* that can be critical to individuals' coping with serious illnesses. It should be noted that the samples in these studies were homogenous, composed primarily of Caucasian middle-class couples; hence, the findings cannot be generalized to more diverse populations.

Psychosocial Interventions to Enhance Couples' Coping With Breast Cancer

Over the last decade there have been several comprehensive reviews of outcome studies on psychosocial interventions for cancer patients (Andersen, 1992; Cwikel, Behar, & Zabora, 1997; Fawzy, Fawzy, Arndt, & Pasnau, 1995; Helgeson & Cohen, 1996; Iacovino & Reesor, 1997; Meyer & Mark, 1995). These reviews cover 76 distinct outcome studies of interventions that included behavioral training, educational groups, individual counseling, and support groups. Although these studies included people with a variety of types of cancer, 64% of the studies included breast cancer patients. Except for a few studies on individual and family counseling, almost all of the studies investigated the effectiveness of peer support groups for patients.

The findings of Spiegel's 1989 study that participation in a therapeutic support group could lengthen the lives of women with metastatic breast cancer led to a proliferation of support groups in the next decade. However, recent studies have questioned the original findings (e.g., Bordeleau et al., 2003; Goodwin et al., 2001). Similarly, Helgeson, Cohen, Schulz, and Yasko (2001) not only found minimal psychosocial benefits of peer support groups for early-stage breast cancer patients but even adverse effects of peer discussion for some subgroups of women. The members of peer support groups had greater intrusive and avoidant thoughts about the illness than the members of comparison groups. Why is support correlated with adjustment in observational studies but not in intervention studies? A few studies suggest that the most important kind of support is emotional support, particularly emotional support that is provided by close family or friends (Dakof & Taylor, 1990; Dunkel-Schetter, 1984; Neuling & Winefield, 1988) and that support from strangers is not the same. Alternately, the time-limited nature of support groups may hinder the transaction of support among members, as the relationship is not as intimate and the support is perceived as artificial in the context of an intervention (Rook & Dooley, 1985). It is possible that longer term peer support interventions may be effective because they foster "real" relationships, transforming an "artificial" relationship into a "natural" one (Helgeson & Cohen, 1996), but there is little empirical evidence for this.

Only seven studies that have included a spouse or significant other have evaluated psychosocial interventions for breast cancer patients (Blanchard, Toseland, & McCallion, 1996; Christensen, 1983; Goldberg & Wool, 1985; Halford, Scott, & Smythe, 2000; Heinrich & Schag, 1985; Sabo, Brown, & Smith, 1986; Samarel & Fawcett, 1992). With the exception of studies by Christensen (1983) and Halford et al. (2000), all of these programs used a therapy group format. The therapy groups either consisted of only spouses without patients (Blanchard et al., 1996; Sabo et al., 1986) or patients with their spouses (Goldberg & Wool, 1985; Heinrich & Schag, 1985; Samarel & Fawcett, 1992).

The intervention studies by Christensen (1983) and Halford et al. (2000) both used randomized group designs. Christensen's intervention involved four counseling sessions with postmastectomy couples and emphasized communication and problem-solving techniques. In the study, 20 postmastectomy patients and their husbands were randomly assigned to the experimental or control (no treatment) condition. Measures of marital happiness, sexual satisfaction, depression, self-esteem, helplessness, anxiety, alienation, and emotional discomfort were administered pretest and posttest (6 weeks after the pretest). Analyses of covariance revealed that both husbands and wives in the treatment group had significantly higher scores on sexual satisfaction than husbands and wives in the control group. Patients who had received the treatment had significantly lower levels of depression than patients in the control group. Also, the husbands who received the treatment had significantly lower levels of discomfort than the husbands who didn't receive the treatment. However, no significant differences were obtained on the other measures. The authors noted that with the small sample, it was difficult to obtain significant results, but these preliminary results provide some promising findings for couple-based interventions.

Halford et al. (2000) conducted a randomized, controlled trial with 90 married women recently diagnosed with early-stage breast or gynecological cancer. Couples were assigned to a couple-based intervention, a cognitive–behavioral educational program, or standard care. The couples-based program, CanCOPE, consisted of an initial session with the cancer patient alone followed by five conjoint sessions with the couple. Data on the effectiveness of the program are currently being analyzed by the authors. Preliminary observations indicate that the treatment was effective and better than individual support provided to the patients alone (Halford et al., 2000).

Although both patients and their partners are affected by the stress of breast cancer, there has been little systematic study of the effectiveness of psychosocial interventions targeted at the couple or examining psychological outcomes for both partners or for the marriage. Given the frequency and intensity of interaction that a patient has with her spouse or partner, psychosocial interventions within an existing relational context may be more effective than peer groups or cognitive behavioral interventions (Radjovic, Nicassio, & Weisman, 1992). Furthermore, current changes in the patterns of medical care transfer greater responsibility from health care professionals to the spouse and the couple, making it all the more important to deal with a couple as a unit and include the partner in treatment plans. For these reasons, a psychosocial intervention for couples facing breast cancer was developed and evaluated. The following section describes the PICP and presents preliminary findings on its effectiveness.

The Partners in Coping Intervention

The development of the PICP was guided by the methods of design and development research for human services (Thomas, 1984) and Barbarin's (1988) clinical work with families coping with childhood cancer. The program was pilot tested with seven couples using a single-subject design (Kayser, 1999). After further revisions, it was tested with 50 couples using a randomized group design.

The conceptual model that guided the design of the PICP is illustrated in Figure 9.1. This model proposes that relationship characteristics, partner support, and quality of dyadic coping are factors that moderate the impact of the stresses of breast cancer on the psychosocial well-being of patients and their partners. The goals of the intervention are to increase the mutual emotional support between partners and patients and to facilitate dyadic coping. Dyadic coping was conceptualized as a process in which partners react to each other's stress signals in order to maintain or return to homeostasis on the individual and couple levels (see chap. 2, this volume; Bodenmann, 1997). Assuming that each partner is willing to invest in the relationship and is committed to the relationship, partners will be motivated to help each other deal with stressful encounters.

DESCRIPTION OF THE PARTNERS IN COPING PROGRAM. The PICP is implemented over nine bi-weekly 1-hour sessions during the first year after the breast cancer diagnosis when the woman is undergoing treatment. (There are

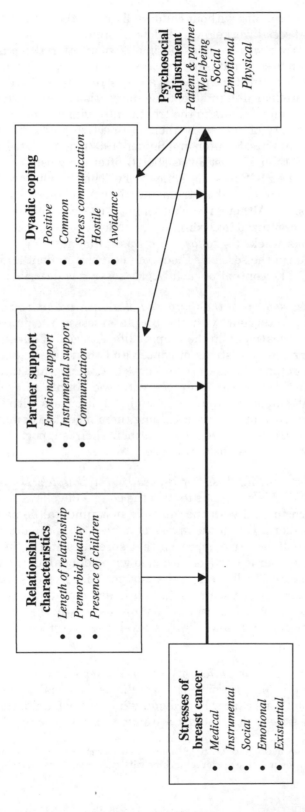

Figure 9.1.   Conceptual model for the development of an intervention for couples coping with breast cancer.

only eight sessions for couples without children living in the home.) The couple meets with a clinical social worker[2] who follows a protocol of specific psychosocial interventions. Work with couples begins as soon after the diagnosis as feasible, that is, when the patient is able to travel to the outpatient clinic at the hospital for the sessions. This time period is a very stressful one in that patients and their partners are learning to accept the diagnosis of cancer, anticipating treatment or making adjustments to the treatment regimen, and beginning to live with the uncertainty of cancer. In their prospective study of newly diagnosed breast cancer patients, Stanton and Snider (1993) found distress and perceived threat were at their highest levels shortly after diagnosis.

Each session of the PICP has a specific theme. The sessions are organized to move from less personal and instrumental issues to more intimate and emotion-focused issues. Although each theme is the central focus of each session, the time is organized according to the following sequence: (a) taking stock of the previous week, (b) follow-up on assignment from the previous session, (c) discussion of the session's theme, and (d) assignment and planning for the next session. The content of each week's session is described next.

Session One: Assessment of the Couple's Relationship and Social Support Network. The initial interview with the couple assesses the impact of the breast cancer and its treatment on the couple's life. A series of questions about how the couple appraises the stress of cancer and their coping behaviors in response to cancer-related stress are discussed. A genogram (McGoldrick, Gerson, & Shellenberger, 1999) is drawn with the couple to identify and describe their social support network. The clinician discusses with the couple the adequacy of their social network in helping them meet the demands of the illness. Suggestions are generated to strengthen their support system and identify specific ways to access help, if needed.

Session Two: Integrating Tasks of Illness Into a Couple's Daily Routine. The overall purpose of this session is to help the couple develop a coordinated, cooperative approach to deal with the multiple instrumental demands of the illness and its treatment. Given the stress of cancer, it is important for the couple to develop a collaborative approach that spreads some of the demands so that one family member is not overburdened with doing all of the work. The clinician asks the couple to list all of the current tasks of the family (e.g., cooking, grocery shopping, housecleaning, and house maintenance) and then identify who does each task. The couple then discusses whether the distribution of these tasks is desirable and effective given the current demands of the cancer on their lives.

Session Three: Caring for Children When a Mother Has Cancer. The clinician assists the couple in assessing their child(ren)'s social and emotional adjustment to the mother's cancer by providing information on developmental issues and signs of stress. Suggestions are made to help the child(ren) deal

---

[2]Although the protocol does not require the practitioner to be a social worker, the clinician should be a mental health practitioner with experience working with cancer patients and familiarity with couples therapy.

with fears and concerns related to their mother's diagnosis and treatment. If the couple has no children, this session is omitted and these couples receive only eight sessions in the program.

Session Four: Personal Coping—Preserving Physical and Psychological Health. This session focuses on helping patients and their partners to identify in themselves and each other their coping style and assess the effectiveness of the way they cope. The goal is to achieve an understanding and respect for each other's way of coping. The clinician facilitates a discussion in which each partner identifies, describes, categorizes, and evaluates the personal coping strategies she or he uses to deal with the emotional strain, existential issues, and practical demands of having cancer or living with a partner with cancer. After an initial discussion of individual coping strategies, the clinician reflects on the couple's dyadic-coping pattern. The couple discusses the effectiveness of and their satisfaction with this coping pattern. The clinician offers suggestions to deal with differences in coping strategies, such as compromising, communicating feelings, giving each other time alone, and reassuring the partner of one's love and concern.

Session Five: Learning New Coping Skills. In this session, the clinician demonstrates relaxation techniques such as focused breathing, guided imagery, and progressive muscle relaxation. She or he helps the couple develop a plan to maintain their physical and emotional health, including such activities as regular exercise, time alone, time to get away from it all, walks, meditation, and use of recreation and leisure opportunities.

Session Six: Enhancing the Couple's Communication. The purpose of this session is to help the couple constructively communicate about the cancer and its treatment. The practitioner teaches the couple specific listening and speaking skills through modeling and role-playing. Emphasis is placed on communicating sensitive disclosures, perspective taking, and empathic listening.

Session Seven: Promoting Supportive Exchanges. This session helps the couple to identify behaviors that each partner perceives as supportive, how to ask for support from one's partner, and how to develop a way that support can be exchanged between partners on a daily basis. The clinician facilitates an exercise based on Caring Days (Stuart, 1980) in which each partner makes a list of supportive and caring behaviors for the other partner to do. After a discussion of each item, the clinician suggests that the couple engage in the behaviors on each other's list during the following weeks and gives them the list to take home.

Session Eight: Enhancing Intimacy and Sexual Functioning. The clinician facilitates a discussion about any changes in the couple's intimacy and sexual functioning since the diagnosis. Information regarding the potential impact of breast cancer treatments on sexual functioning is shared. The clinician teaches skills in dealing with changes in sexual functioning, assists the couple in openly communicating any concerns around sexuality, and suggests alternative ways of expressing intimacy.

Session Nine: Living With Cancer. The goal of this session is to help the couple move from a pattern of adaptation that is crisis oriented to one that attempts to incorporate the illness into their daily lives. It involves the acceptance of the fact that life will never be exactly the same as it was before the diagnosis but challenges them to define what a "normal" life for them as a couple can be. This may be a new "normal" pattern of life or it could be their prediagnosis "normal" life.

EFFICACY OF THE PARTNERS IN COPING PROGRAM: A PRELIMINARY TRIAL. The study used a randomized group design with 50 couples in which one partner had breast cancer, and couples were randomly assigned to the PICP or received standard services (SS) offered at the hospital where they were being treated. Couples assigned to the SS condition were provided with the name and telephone number of a social worker at the hospital who was available for individual counseling, family counseling, crisis intervention, community referrals, tangible assistance, and discharge planning on the patient's request. Patients who had received a diagnosis of primary nonmetastatic breast cancer within the last 3 months and were currently receiving treatment such as chemotherapy, radiation, or a combination of treatments were eligible for participation. In addition, the patient had to be married or in an intimate relationship.

Before randomization to treatment, couples completed questionnaires assessing their adjustment to the cancer: the Functional Assessment of Cancer Therapy Scale (FACT-B; Cella et al., 1993), the Quality of Life Scale—Spouse Version (Ebbesen, Guyatt, McCartney, & Oldridge, 1990), and the Illness Intrusiveness Scale (Devins, Hunsley, Mandlin, Taub, & Paul, 1997). Dyadic coping was measured by Bodenmann's (1997) Dyadic Coping Scale, which consists of five types of coping: (a) common dyadic coping (both partners are participating in the coping more or less symmetrically in order to handle stress); (b) positive coping (partners are supporting each other in coping efforts); (c) stress communication (partners are openly communicating about their stress to each other); (d) hostile coping (support is accompanied by disparagement, mocking, sarcasm, or minimizing the seriousness of the partner's stress); and (e) avoidance (one partner is withdrawing or distancing her- or himself from the partner to avoid dealing with stress). Emotional support was measured by the Mutuality Psychological Development Questionnaire (MPDQ; Genero, Miller, Surrey, & Baldwin, 1992). The questionnaires were given when couples were enrolled in the study (Time 1), 6 months postbaseline (Time 2), and 1 year postbaseline (Time 3).

The sample was quite homogenous—middle-class, White (90%), and highly educated (89% had a college or postgraduate education). Ninety percent of the couples were married and there was one lesbian couple. The average age of the patients was 47 years, and the average age of the partners was 49 years. Couples had been either married or living together for an average of 21 years, although there was a wide range (1–41 years) and most (78%) had children. The patients assigned to the two conditions did not differ on the types of medical treatment they were receiving or on any of the sociodemographic variables.

To determine the effects of the PICP on the patients' and partners' well-being and relationship functioning, repeated measures analyses of variance

(ANOVAs) were performed. Group (PICP or SS) was the between-subjects factor, and time (Time 1, 2, or 3) was the within-subjects factor. An overall Group × Time interaction in the predicted direction would indicate treatment effects. Separate ANOVAs were performed for patients and partners on well-being and relationship measures.

Individual Well-Being. There was a trend toward a significant Group × Time interaction on patient well-being, $F(1, 42) = 3.31$, $p < .08$, but no effect for partners. As shown in Figure 9.2, PICP patients' mean scores on overall well-being increased over time. Although patients in the SS group also improved, the change was not as dramatic as for the patients in the PICP.

Relationship Functioning. For patients, the effect for common dyadic coping approached significance, $F(1, 42) = 3.27$, $p < .08$, and the effect was in the predicted direction. Over time, patients in the PICP group had significantly higher means on common dyadic coping than patients in the SS group (see Figure 9.3). No Group × Time interaction effects were found with the other four types of dyadic coping.

Significant Group × Time interaction effects were found for the partners on one of the types of dyadic coping, and trend effects were found for two other types of coping. Partners who received the PICP had significantly higher means on stress communication coping $F(1, 40) = 3.54$, $p < .04$. As shown in Figure 9.4, PICP partners were more willing to communicate their own stress to their wives than were partners who received SS. The interactions for the two negative forms of dyadic coping approached significance, with $F(1, 40) = 3.54$, $p < .07$ for avoidance coping and $F(1, 40) = 3.27$, $p < .08$ for hostile coping. Over

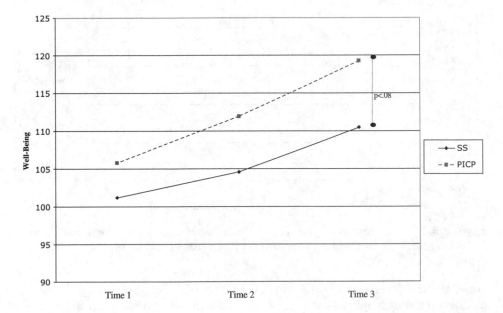

Figure 9.2. Comparison of breast cancer patients in standard services (SS) and Partners in Coping Program (PICP) on well-being across three times.

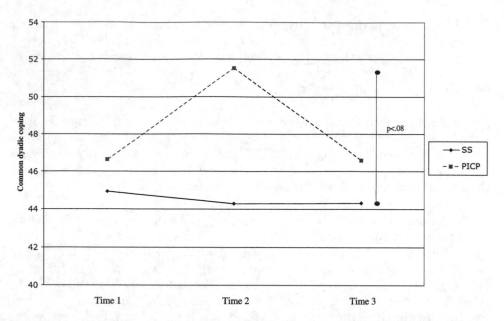

Figure 9.3.   Comparison of patients in standard services (SS) and Partners in Coping Program (PICP) on common dyadic coping across three times.

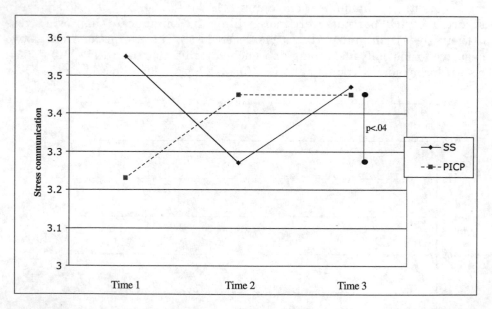

Figure 9.4.   Comparison of partners of breast cancer patients in standard services (SS) and Partners in Coping Program (PICP) on stress communication across three times.

time, the PICP partners had lower scores on avoidance coping (see Figure 9.5) or hostile dyadic coping (see Figure 9.6) than those who received SS.

No significant Group × Time interaction effects were found for either patients or partners on the measure of emotional support. In general, the

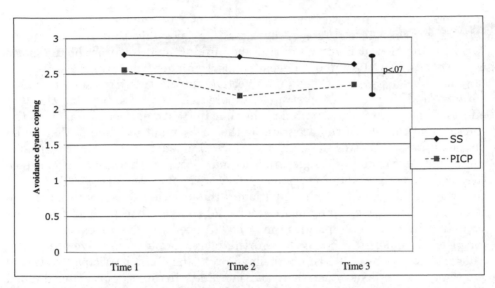

Figure 9.5. Comparison of partners of breast cancer patients in standard services (SS) and Partners in Coping Program (PICP) on avoidance dyadic coping across three times.

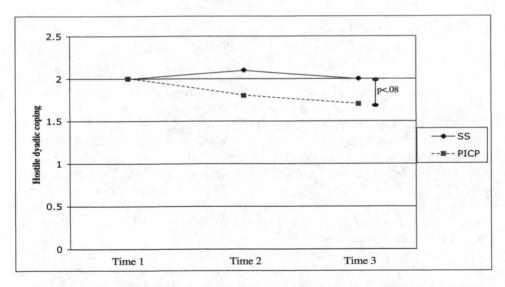

Figure 9.6. Comparison of partners of breast cancer patients in standard services (SS) and Partners in Coping Program (PICP) on hostile dyadic coping across three times.

scores on emotional support were at high levels at baseline, and this may have contributed to the lack of change in them over time.

The breast cancer patients who participated in the PICP evaluated their dyadic coping as involving more common dyadic coping at Time 2 (6 months postbaseline). This indicates that the intervention may have facilitated a sense of *we-ness* in coping with the illness. Unfortunately, the gains in common dyadic coping were not maintained, as was evidenced by a return to couples' baseline levels 12 months later. It is possible that the treatment regimen was most demanding during the initial 6 months after the diagnosis and leveled off by the end of the year. Thus, common dyadic coping strategies may have been greatly needed (and effective) during the first 6 months after surgery, and then use of the strategy tapered off. It is also possible that the effects of the program are limited to the time in treatment because most of the couples had completed the program by the assessment at Time 2. Continued participation or booster sessions may have helped to maintain the use of common dyadic coping strategies. Indeed, many couples therapy programs face the challenge of maintaining results.

Many of the effects of participation in the program were centered on the reduction of negative coping or interpersonal communication behaviors. Participating in a biweekly program may have raised the awareness and monitoring of these negative behaviors. Furthermore, couples may have been more reluctant to use negative coping behaviors during their participation in the program. Discussions with their partner and therapist may have helped people to gain a higher level of empathy for their partner, which facilitated more supportive coping behaviors and fewer negative behaviors. However, we still need to explore the reasons for the tendency for coping behaviors to return closer to the baseline measures at Time 3.

Future Directions

There is a clear need for empirically based interventions for couples coping with breast cancer. A growing body of research supports the propositions that breast cancer patients do not cope alone but with their partners (Hannum et al., 1991; Kuijer et al., 2000; Pistrang, Barker, & Rutter, 1997; Ptacek et al., 1994; Skerrett, 1998; Weiss, 2004; Zunkel, 2002) and that the mutual support between patients and partners has an impact on the positive adjustment of both people (Kayser & Sormanti, 2002, Kayser et al., 1999; Northouse et al., 2001). Although couples-based interventions may facilitate support and dyadic coping, how these psychosocial interventions should be delivered, at what point in the illness and treatment they should be delivered, and how long they should continue remain as future challenges.

Several obstacles hinder couples from participating fully in a program such as the PICP. These include distance from cancer hospitals, work schedules, and childcare responsibilities. Interventions delivered through the Internet, by the telephone, or through local community-based agencies and outpatient health clinics may be viable alternatives.

The PICP was developed for couples early in the process of coping with breast cancer but should be tested with other populations. For example, it could be adapted for patients with metastatic disease. Some research indicates that relationship quality and partners' coping are significantly related to patients' emotional well-being (Giese-Davis, Hermanson, Koopman, Weibel, & Spiegel, 2000). Thus, although the content may need to be changed—for example, adding sessions on existential issues around death and dying—the basic format and emphasis on dyadic coping and interpersonal communication could remain.

Although the PICP showed promising results for a sample of middle-class and White couples, we do not know if results would be similar for a group of non-White or working-class couples. A larger trial is needed to allow for greater generalization. In a similar vein, the intervention needs a better test with lesbian couples. Lesbian women are at a slightly higher risk for developing breast cancer than heterosexual women (Torassa, 2002). However, health care services may not be attuned to the relationships issues and other social issues unique to lesbian patients or couples (Perry & O'Hanlan, 1998).

Given the variety of stresses and the heightened level of stress associated with breast cancer, a dyadic approach to therapy offers great promise. Although the diagnosis elicits feelings of loss, hopelessness, and vulnerability, it also presents an opportunity for psychological growth. The PICP builds on couples' strengths, transforming an otherwise painful experience into one in which each person grows through the connection with the other.

References

American Cancer Society. (2002). *Breast Cancer Facts & Figures 2001–2002*. Retrieved July 3, 2003, from http://www.cancer.org/downloads/STT/BrCaFF2001.pdf

Anderson, B. (1992). Psychological interventions for cancer patients. *Journal of Consulting and Clinical Psychology, 60*, 552–568.

Anderson, B. (1994). Surviving cancer. *Cancer, 74*(Suppl. 4), 1484–1495.

Barbarin, O. (1988). *Childhood cancer project treatment manual*. Unpublished manuscript, University of Michigan, Ann Arbor.

Baum, A., & Posluszny, D. M. (2001). Traumatic stress as a target for intervention with cancer patients. In A. Baum & B. L. Andersen (Eds.), *Psychosocial interventions for cancer* (pp. 143–174). Washington, DC: American Psychological Association.

Blanchard C., Toseland R., & McCallion, P. (1996). The effects of a problem-solving intervention with spouses of cancer patients. *Journal of Psychosocial Oncology, 14*(2), 1–21.

Bloom, J. R. (1982). Social support, accommodation to stress and adjustment to breast cancer. *Social Science Medicine, 16*, 1329–1338.

Bloom, J. R., & Spiegel, D. (1984). The relationship of two dimensions of social support to the psychological well-being and social functioning of women with advanced breast cancer. *Social Science Medicine, 19*, 831–837.

Bodenmann, G. (1997). Dyadic coping—a systemic-transactional view of stress and coping among couples: Theory and empirical findings. *European Review of Applied Psychology, 47*, 137–140.

Bordeleau, L., Szalai, J. P., Ennis, M., Leszcz, M., Speca, M., Sela, R., et al. (2003). Quality of life in a randomized trial of group psychosocial support in metastatic breast cancer: Overall effects of the intervention and an exploration of missing data. *Journal of Clinical Oncology, 21*, 1944–1951.

Cella, D. F., Tulsky, D. S., Gray, G., Sarafian, B., Linn, E., Bonomi, A., et al. (1993). The Functional Assessment of Cancer Therapy Scale: Development and validation of the general measure. *Journal of Clinical Oncology, 11*, 570–579.

Charles, K., Sellick, S. M., Montesanto, B., & Mohide, E. A. (1996). Priorities of cancer survivors regarding psychosocial needs. *Journal of Psychosocial Oncology, 13*, 1–22.

Chesler, M. A., & Barbarin, O. A. (1986). *Childhood cancer and the family: Meeting the challenge of stress and support*. New York: Brunner/Mazel.

Christensen, D. (1983). Postmastectomy couple counseling: An outcome study of a tructured treatment protocol. *Journal of Sex & Marital Therapy, 9*, 266–275.

Collins, R. L., Taylor, S. E., & Skokan, L. A. (1990). A better world or a shattered vision? Changes in life perspectives following victimization. *Social Cognition, 8*, 263–285.

Cordova, M. J., Andrykowski, M. A., Kenady, D. E., McGrath, P. C., Sloan, D. A., & Redd, W. H. (1995). Frequency and correlates of posttraumatic-stress-disorder-like symptoms after treatment for breast cancer, *Journal of Consulting and Clinical Psychology, 63,* 981–986.

Cutrona, C. E. (1996). *Social support in couples.* Thousand Oaks, CA: Sage.

Cwikel, J. G., Behar, L. C., Zabora, J. R. (1997). Psychosocial factors that affect the survival of adult cancer patients: A review of research. *Journal of Psychosocial Oncology, 15*(3/4), 1–34.

Dakof, G. A., & Taylor, S. E. (1990). Victims' perceptions of social support: What is helpful from whom? *Journal of Personality and Social Psychology, 58,* 80–89.

Devins, G. M., Hunsley, J., Mandlin, H. Taub, K. J., & Paul, L. C. (1997). The marital context of end-stage renal disease: Illness intrusiveness and perceived changes in family environment, *Annals of Behavioral Medicine, 19*(4), 325–332.

Dunkel-Schetter, C. (1984). Social support and cancer: Findings based on patient interviews and their implications. *Journal of Social Issues, 40,* 77–98.

Ebbesen, L. S., Guyatt, G. H., McCartney, N., & Oldridge, N. B. (1990). Measuring quality of life in cardiac spouses. *Journal of Epidemiology, 43,* 481–487.

Ell, K., Nishimoto, R., Mediansky, K., Mantell, J., & Hamovitch, M. (1992). Social relations, social support and survival among patients with cancer. *Journal of Psychosomatic Research, 36,* 531–541.

Fawzy, I., Fawzy, N. W., Arndt, L. A., & Pasnau, R. O. (1995). Critical review of psychosocial interventions in cancer care. *Archives of General Psychiatry, 52,* 100–113.

Genero, N. P., Miller, J. B., Surrey, J., Baldwin, L. (1992). Measuring perceived mutuality in close relationships: Validation of the Mutual Psychological Development Questionnaire. *Journal of Family Psychology, 6*(1), 36–48.

Germino, B. B., Fife, B., & Funk, S. G. (1995). Cancer and the partner relationship: What is its meaning? *Seminars in Oncology Nursing, 11,* 43–50.

Giese-Davis, J., Hermanson, K., Koopman, C., Weibel, D., & Spiegel, D. (2000). Quality of couples' relationship and adjustment to metastatic breast cancer. *Journal of Family Psychology, 14,* 251–266.

Goldberg, R. J., & Wool, M. S. (1985). Psychotherapy for the spouses of lung cancer patients: Assessment of an intervention. *Psychotherapy Psychosomatics, 43,* 141–150.

Goodwin, P. J., Leszcz, M., Ennis, M., Koopmans, J., Vincent, L., Guther, H., et al. (2001). The effect of group psychosocial support on survival in metastatic breast cancer. *New England Journal of Medicine, 345,* 1719–1726.

Greenberg, D. B., Goorin, A., Gebhart, M. C., Gupta, L., Stier, N., Harmon, D., & Mankin, H. (1994). Quality of life in osteosarcoma survivors. *Oncology, 8*(11), 19–25.

Halford, W. K., Scott, J. L., & Smythe, J. (2000). Couples and coping with cancer: Helping each other through the night. In K. B. Schmaling & T. G. Sher (Eds.), *The psychology of couples and illness: Theory, research, and practice* (pp. 135–170). Washington, DC: American Psychological Association.

Hannum, J. W., Giese-Davis, J., Harding, K., & Hatfield, A. K. (1991). Effects of individual and marital variables on coping with cancer. *Journal of Psychosocial Oncology, 9,* 1–20.

Harwood, K. V., & O'Connor, A. P. (1994). Sexuality and breast cancer: Overview of issues. *Innovations in Oncology Nursing, 10*(23), 30–33, 51.

Heinrich, R. L., & Schag, C. C. (1985). Stress and activity management: Group treatment for cancer patients and spouses. *Journal of Consulting and Clinical Psychology, 53,* 439–446.

Helgeson, V., & Cohen, S. (1996). Social support and adjustment to cancer: Reconciling descriptive, correlational, and intervention research. *Health Psychology, 15*(2), 132–148.

Helgeson, V. S., Cohen, S., Schulz, R., & Yasko, J. (2001). Group support interventions for people with cancer: Benefits and hazards. In A. Baum & B. L. Andersen (Eds.), *Psychosocial interventions for cancer* (pp. 269–286). Washington, DC: American Psychological Association.

Helgeson, V. S., Snyder, P., & Seltman, H. (2004). Psychological and physical adjustment to breast cancer over 4 years: Identifying distinct trajectories of change. *Health Psychology, 23,* 3–15.

Hoskins, C. N., Baker, S., Budin, W., Ekstrom, D., Maislin, G., Sherman, D., et al. (1996). Adjustment among husbands of women with breast cancer. *Journal of Psychosocial Oncology, 14*(1) 41–69.

Iacovino, V., & Reesor, K. (1997). Literature on intervention to address cancer patients' psychosocial needs: What does it tell us? *Journal of Psychosocial Oncology, 15*(2), 47–71.

Irvine, D., Brown, B., Crooks, D., Roberts, J., & Browne, G. (1991). Psychosocial adjustment in women with breast cancer. *Cancer, 67,* 1097.

Kayser, K. (1999, November). *The development and testing of a psychosocial program for breast cancer patients and their partners.* Paper presented at the 61st Annual Conference of the National Council on Family Relations, Irvine, CA.

Kayser, K., & Sormanti, M. (2002). A follow-up study of women with cancer: Their psychosocial well-being and close relationships. *Social Work in Health Care, 35,* 391–406.

Kayser, K., Sormanti, M., & Strainchamps, E. (1999). Women coping with cancer: The impact of close relationships on psychosocial adjustment. *Psychology of Women Quarterly, 23,* 725–739.

Kuijer, R. G., Ybema, J. F., Buunk, B. P., DeJong, G. M., Thijs-Boer, F., & Sanderman, R. (2000). Active engagement, protective buffering, and overprotection: Three ways of giving support by intimate partners of patients with cancer. *Journal of Social and Clinical Psychology, 19,* 256–275.

Lewis, F. M., Woods, N. F., Hough, E. E., & Bensley, L. S. (1989). The family's functioning with chronic illness in the mother: The spouse's perspective. *Social Science and Medicine, 29,* 1261–1269.

Lichtman, R. R., Taylor, S. E., & Wood, J. V. (1987). Social support and marital adjustment after breast cancer. *Journal of Psychosocial Oncology, 5*(3), 47–74.

Maguire, P. (1981). The repercussions of mastectomy on the family. *International Journal of Family Psychiatry, 1,* 485–503.

Manne, S. L. (1998). Cancer in the marital context: A review of the literature. *Cancer Investigation, 16,* 188–202.

Manne, S. L. (1999). Intrusive thoughts and psychological distress among cancer patients: The role of spouse avoidance and criticism, *Journal of Consulting and Clinical Psychology, 67,* 539–546.

Massie, M. J., & Holland, J. C. (1991). Psychological reactions to breast cancer in the pre- and postsurgical treatment period. *Seminars in Surgical Oncology, 7,* 320.

McGoldrick, M., Gerson, R., & Shellenberger, S. (1999). *Genograms: Assessment and intervention* (2nd ed.). New York: Norton.

Meyer, T., & Mark, M. (1995). Effects of psychosocial interventions with adult cancer patients: A meta-analysis of randomized experiments. *Health Psychology, 14*(2), 101–108.

Meyerowitz, B. E. (1983). Postmastectomy coping strategies and quality of life. *Health Psychology, 2,* 117–132.

Meyerowitz, B. E. (1986). Psychosocial correlates of breast cancer and its treatment. *Psychological Bulletin, 99,* 108–131.

Morse, S. R., & Fife, B. (1998). Coping with a partner's cancer: Adjustment at four stages of the illness trajectory. *Oncology Nursing Forum, 25,* 751–760.

Nadeau, J. W. (1998). *Families making sense of death.* Thousand Oaks, CA: Sage.

Neuling, S. J., & Winefield, H. R. (1988). Social support and recovery after surgery for breast cancer: Frequency and correlates of supportive behaviours by family, friends and surgeon. *Social Science Medicine, 27,* 385–391.

Northouse, L. L. (1989). A longitudinal study of the adjustment of patients and husbands to breast cancer. *Oncology Nursing Forum, 16,* 511–516.

Northouse, L. L., Dorris, G., & Charron-Moore, C. (1995). Factors affecting couples' adjustment to recurrent breast cancer. *Nursing Research, 37,* 91–95.

Northouse, L. L., & Swain, M. A. (1987). Adjustment of patients and husbands to the initial impact of breast cancer, *Nursing Research, 36,* 221–225.

Northouse, L. L., Templin, T., & Mood, D. (2001). Couples' adjustment to breast disease during the first year following diagnosis. *Journal of Behavioral Medicine, 24,* 115–136.

Northouse, L. L., Templin, T., Mood, D., & Oberst, M. (1998). Couples' adjustment to breast cancer and benign breast disease: A longitudinal analysis. *Psycho-Oncology, 7,* 37–48.

Nuehring, E. M., & Barr, W. E. (1980). Mastectomy: Impact on patients and families. *Health and Social Work, 5,* 51–58.

Oberst, M. T., & James, R. H. (1985). Going home: Patient and spouse adjustment following cancer surgery. *Topics in Clinical Nursing, 7,* 46–57.

Omne-Ponten, M., Holmberg, L., & Sjoden, P. O. (1994). Psychosocial adjustment among women with breast cancer Stages I and II: Six-year follow-up of consecutive patients. *Journal of Clinical Oncology, 12,* 1778–1782.

Penman, D. T., Bloom, J. R., Fotopoulos, S., Cook, M. R., Holland, J. C., Gates, C., et al. (1986). The impact of mastectomy on self-concept and social function: A combined cross-sectional and longitudinal study with comparison groups. *Women and Health, 12,* 101–130.

Perry, M. J., & O'Hanlan, K. A. (1998). Lesbian health. In E. A. Blechman & K. D. Brownell (Eds.), *Behavioral medicine and women: A comprehensive handbook* (pp. 843–848). New York: Guilford.

Pistrang, N., & Barker, C. (1995). The partner relationship in psychological response to breast cancer. *Social Science and Medicine, 40,* 789–797.

Pistrang, N., Barker, C., & Rutter, C. (1997). Social support as conversation: Analysing breast cancer patients' interactions with their partners. *Social Science and Medicine, 45,* 773–782.

Polinsky, M. L. (1994). Functional status of long-term breast cancer survivors: Demonstrating chronicity. *Health and Social Work, 19*(3), 165–173.

Primomo, J., Yates, B. C., & Woods, N. F. (1990). Social support for women during chronic illness: The relationship among sources and types to adjustment. *Research in Nursing and Health, 13,* 153–161.

Ptacek, J. T., Ptacek, J. J., & Dodge, K. L. (1994). Coping with breast cancer from the perspectives of husbands and wives. *Journal of Psychosocial Oncology, 12,* 47–72.

Radjovic, V., Nicassio, P. M., & Weisman, M. H. (1992). Behavioral intervention with and without family support for rheumatoid arthritis. *Behavior Therapy, 23,* 13–30.

Rolland, J. S. (1994). *Families, illness, and disability: An integrative model.* New York: Basic Books

Rook, K. S., & Dooley, D. (1985). Applying social support research: Theoretical problems and future directions. *Journal of Social Issues, 41,* 5–28.

Sabo, D. (1990). Men, death anxiety, and denial: Critical feminist interpretations of adjustment to mastectomy. In C. Clark, F. Fritz, & P. Rieder (Eds.), *Clinical sociological perspectives on illness and loss* (pp. 71–84). Philadelphia: Charles Press.

Sabo, D., Brown, J., & Smith, C. (1986). The male role and mastectomy: Support groups and men's adjustment. *Journal of Psychosocial Oncology, 4*(1/2), 19–31.

Samarel, N., & Fawcett, J. (1992). Enhancing adaptation to breast cancer: The addition of coaching to support groups. *Oncology Nursing Forum, 19,* 591–596.

Schain, W. S. (1988). The sexual and intimate consequences of breast cancer treatment. *CA: A Cancer Journal for Clinicians, 38,* 154–161.

Skerrett, K. (1998). Couple adjustment to the experience of breast cancer. *Families, Systems & Health, 16,* 281–298.

Slaikeu, R. (1990). *Crisis intervention: A handbook for practice and research.* Boston: Allyn & Bacon.

Spiegel, D. (1995). Essentials of psychotherapeutic intervention for cancer patients. *Support Care Cancer, 3,* 252–256.

Spiegel, D. (1996). Cancer and depression. *British Journal of Psychiatry, 30*(Suppl.), 109.

Spiegel, D., Bloom, J. R., Kraemer, H. C., & Gottheil, E. (1989). Effect of psychosocial treatment on survival of patients with metastatic breast cancer. *Lancet, 2,* 888–891.

Stanton, A. L., & Snider, P. R. (1993). Coping with a breast cancer diagnosis: A prospective study. *Health Psychology, 12,* 16–23.

Stuart, R. B. (1980). *Helping couples change: A social learning approach to marital therapy.* New York: Guilford Press.

Taylor, S. E. (1983). Adjustment to threatening events: A theory of cognitive adaptation. *American Psychologist, 38,* 1161–1173.

Thomas, E. J. (1984). *Designing interventions for the helping professions.* Beverly Hills, CA: Sage.

Torassa, U. (2002, April 28). Higher breast cancer risk for lesbians not borne out, study finds. *San Francisco Chronicle.* Retrieved July 1, 2003, from http://www.sfgate.com/cgi-bin/article.cgi?file=/chronicle/archive/2002

Walker, B. L. (1997). Adjustment of husbands and wives to breast cancer. *Cancer Practice, 5*(2), 92–98.

Weiss, T. (2004). Correlates of posttraumatic growth in husbands of breast cancer survivors, *Psycho-Oncology, 13,* 260–268.

Zunkel, G. (2002). Relational coping processes: Couples' response to a diagnosis of early stage breast cancer. *Journal of Psychosocial Oncology, 20(4),* 39–55.

Author Index

Numbers in italics refer to entries in the reference sections.

Subject Index

ABCX model, 14
Acceptance, Rogerian helping component, 101–102
Accommodation
  determinants, 59–60
  social support difference, 79–80, 88
  in stepfamilies, 60
"Active engagement" coping, 36
Active listening, 169
Acute stress
  chronic stress interactions, 15–17, 28–31
  contextual effects, 15–17, 28–31
  Life Experiences Survey measure, 21–22
  longitudinal study, newlyweds, 20–30
  marital satisfaction changes, newlyweds, 23–30
  measurement, 21–22
Ambivalent dyadic coping
  couples intervention effect, 170–171
  description of, 39
Anger, 63. See also Confrontation
Anxious–ambivalent attachment
  and causal attributions, 88
  and perceived social support, 77–78
    case illustration, 86–87
Atherosclerosis, and marital quality, 84
Attachment orientation
  and causal attributions, 88
  intervention implications, 89
  and social support attributions, 75, 77–78
    case illustrations, 85–87
  trust effects of, 82–83, 88
Attributions. See Causal attributions
Avoidance coping, breast cancer, 187–189
Avoidant attachment
  and causal attributions, 88
  and perceived social support, 77–78
    case illustration, 86

Background stressors, and acute stress, 15–17
Bible Belt states
  high divorce rate, 13–14, 30–31
  socioeconomic stressors in, 14, 30–31
Bonding, and helping interactions, 102
Breast cancer, 175–191
  avoidance coping, 178
  coping behaviors, 179
  and division of household labor, 151
  emotional stressors, 176–177
  emotional support role, 177–179
  helping interactions analysis, 106–109

medical stressors, 176
partner's adjustment, 179–180
Partners in Coping Intervention, 182–191
  efficacy, 186–190
peer support groups, 181
"problematic couples," 180
Brief COPE, 130–131
Brief Ways of Coping scale, 58

Cancer, 146. See also Breast cancer
CanCOPE program, 182
Cardiovascular disease
  marital quality link, 84
  protective buffering in, 139–140
Caregiver coping
  gender differences, 145–153
  gender gap, 149–153
Caring Days exercise, 185
Causal attributions
  and attachment orientation, 88
  intervention implications, 89
  and perceived social support, 75–77, 87–90
  trust association, 81–82, 88
Child care, caregiver gender gap, 151
Child misbehavior, stepfamily coping, 61
Chronic illness
  caregiver coping, gender differences, 145–153
  division of household labor, 149–153
  gender differences in coping, 129–131, 137–153
  individual versus relationship coping, 125–127
  relationship awareness in, 121–134
Chronic stress
  acute stress interactions, 15–17, 28–31
  contextual effects, 15–17, 28–31
  longitudinal study, newlyweds, 20–30
  marital functioning effects, 44–45
  marital satisfaction changes, newlyweds, 23–30
  measurement, 22–23
Cognitive–behavioral techniques, 165
Common dyadic coping
  couples intervention effect, 170
  description of, 38–39
  and marital satisfaction, 44
Communication training. See also Stress communication
  breast cancer intervention, 187
  in Couples Coping Enhancement Training, 161, 166, 169–170

About the Editors

Tracey A. Revenson, PhD, is a professor of psychology at The Graduate Center of The City University of New York. She is the coauthor of *Understanding Rheumatoid Arthritis* (1996) and *A Piaget Primer: How a Child Thinks* (1996) and the coeditor of the *Handbook of Health Psychology* (2001), *A Quarter Century of Community Psychology* (2002), and *Ecological Research to Promote Social Change* (2002). She was the founding editor-in-chief of the journal *Women's Health: Research on Gender, Behavior and Policy.* Dr. Revenson is well-known for her research on stress and coping processes among individuals, couples, and families facing chronic physical illness and the influence of interpersonal relationships on health. She was awarded a Senior International Fellowship from the Fogarty International Center at the National Institutes of Health to study cross-cultural issues in coping with chronic illness. She is the current president of Division 38 (Health Psychology) of the American Psychological Association.

Karen Kayser, PhD, is a professor in the Graduate School of Social Work at Boston College. She received her MSW degree and her PhD in social work and psychology from the University of Michigan and completed a National Institute on Child Health and Human Development postdoctoral fellowship in the area of families coping with childhood cancer at the University of Michigan. She has published books and articles in the areas of marital disaffection, stress and coping, intervention research, and couples therapy. Dr. Kayser has received grants from the American Cancer Society and the Massachusetts Department of Public Health Breast Cancer Research Program for her research on women and cancer. She has written and lectured extensively on couples coping with breast cancer and recently has completed a clinical research study of an innovative couples psychosocial intervention at the Dana-Farber Cancer Institute and Massachusetts General Hospital in Boston.

Guy Bodenmann, PhD, is an associate professor of clinical psychology at the University of Fribourg, Switzerland, and the director of the Institute for Family Research and Counseling. He studied at the University of Berne and the University of Fribourg in Switzerland as well as the University of Washington, Seattle. His main research topics are stress and coping in couples, the prediction of marital decline and divorce, prevention of marital distress, marital therapy, and depression in marriage. He is a cognitive–behavioral therapist who specializes in the field of marital therapy. He developed the Couple's Coping Enhancement Training, a marital distress prevention program based on stress and coping research in close relationships.